D0408321

THE LIVING ROOM

THE LIVING ROOM

A LUNG CANCER COMMUNITY OF COURAGE

BONNIE J. ADDARIO
WITH JON LAND

Post Hill
PRESS

A POST HILL PRESS BOOK

The Living Room:
A Lung Cancer Community of Courage
© 2021 by Bonnie J. Addario
All Rights Reserved

ISBN: 978-1-64293-736-7
ISBN (eBook): 978-1-64293-737-4

Cover art by Sheila von Driska, White Space
Interior design and composition by Greg Johnson, Textbook Perfect

Post Hill Press
New York • Nashville
posthillpress.com

Published in the United States of America
1 2 3 4 5 6 7 8 9 10

To my family,
Tony, Danielle, Andrea and Jared, et al,
for joining the fight to end lung cancer.

CONTENTS

If you're passionate about an injustice,
then do something about it.

—ROBERT F. KENNEDY

FOREWORD

By Kristie L. Kahl
Editorial Director,

cure

Hope. Hope is defined as an optimistic state of mind, with the expectation of positive outcomes in respect to circumstances or an event in one's life.

This is a word I hear often at CURE®, which stands for Cancer Updates, Research, and Education. CURE® works with countless patients, caregivers, advocates, and health care professionals—all with that common theme: hope. Hope that there will one day be a cure. Hope that we get more people screened to prevent this terrible disease from being found too late. Hope that we continue to treat individuals long term, so that they can live with the disease with improved quality of life. Hope that there are major breakthroughs just ahead on the horizon. Hope that fewer and fewer people have to hear those three little words: "You have cancer."

There is much hope for the future of cancer and its treatment. And it is with individuals like Bonnie J. Addario, and foundations like the GO2 Foundation, that we can offer hope to many. In particular, such hope is seen throughout the lung cancer community.

We were delighted when we heard Bonnie and Jon were creating this book. A book of hope. A book full of courageous journeys. A book that shows community at its core. A book that gives many a voice, a platform to share their story. At CURE®, we have a community of patients who share their stories regularly as well. It is their courage that helps others realize they are not alone in their own cancer journey.

Thriving with Hope

A recent story of hope that sticks out in my mind is from Emily Bennett Taylor, a newlywed when she received a stage IV lung cancer diagnosis in 2012. She decided to stay positive and have the upper hand against cancer. Wanting a family and keeping in mind that happy times would follow the dark days, the pair used a surrogate and welcomed twin daughters—one being named Hope. "Hope" was a word often used during her treatment, and Emily was also treated at City of Hope Medical Center. People can find Emily through her blog, Emily Kicks Cancer.

"We originally created that site as a way to keep everyone informed about how I was doing with treatments," she said. "Now it's a way to offer hope to others. When I was diagnosed, there weren't a lot of positive stories about people surviving this type of cancer. I want to change that and inspire others to seek out the best medical care so they can fulfill their life dreams."

Another survivor, Susan Warmerdam—who was forty-seven when she received her stage IV lung cancer diagnosis—found hope in a clinical trial. Her tumor test showed EGFR and KRAS mutations, allowing her to join a clinical trial for an experimental drug as a first-line treatment for lung cancer. Admittedly reluctant at first, she went on to note that if it weren't for other people with the courage to join a trial before her, she wouldn't have been afforded the opportunity. "You never know when the next new drug will be the miracle cure."

"When people come to me for advice, I tell them I am proof that a lung cancer diagnosis is not a death sentence. Stay positive and hopeful because the next drug you need may be right around the corner,"

Warmerdam said. "But you have to educate yourself so that you can be your own best advocate."

Seeing the Good in Bad

One aspect of hope is the ability to see the good in a bad situation. For example, in an episode on the "CURE Talks Cancer" podcast, we spoke with Dr. Dan Tran, an oral and maxillofacial surgeon at Virginia Commonwealth University, who received a stage IV lung cancer diagnosis at the age of thirty. Three years out from his diagnosis, Tran discussed what his journey was like and what advice he offered others. One aspect he holds highest: controlling what he could throughout his diagnosis and treatment.

"Everyone gets dealt a different set of cards, and I got dealt a crappy hand," said Tran. "But it kind of depends on what you do with it. I've always had a pretty laid-back kind of personality and understood that there's things that I can control and things I can't control. This is something I could not control, but I can control what I do with it."

When I first started at CURE®, one of the first survivors I spoke with was Taylor Bell Duck—a young division I college soccer player diagnosed at the age of twenty-one who has since worked to raise awareness about lung cancer and serves as an ambassador for Your Cancer Game Plan. I spoke with her as she celebrated her ten-year "cancer-versary." I remember most her positive outlook, embracing her new life, and how others can relish the big victories of everyday life—big and small.

"Celebrate big and do the things that you love," she said. "It is important to have a day to celebrate your life, and the journey patients go through is so important...so go eat cupcakes and have champagne!" I will admit, she is the reason I always remember to eat the cupcakes!

It is what you do with your diagnosis that makes a difference. I've been so inspired over the years, hearing from so many about how they see their diagnosis as a "glass-half-full" situation. Another patient I've spoken with, Ashley Stringer, has made it a point to make the little moments count since her diagnosis. Ashley was diagnosed with lung cancer at the age of thirty-four—something that took her by complete shock as a young never-smoker. As a young mother, she made an effort to continue to exercise and change her diet. Moreover, she cherishes her faith and leans on friends, family, and coworkers for support—cherishing her time now more than ever before.

"I think until you've been put in a position that I'm in, we sometimes tend to take our lives and time that we have for granted," she said. "And so that's something that, once I received the diagnosis, I really was trying to make sure that I make the most of my time. Whatever time I have left and being intentional with the time I do have and spending time with my kids and my husband and just really making the little moments count."

It is with these positive outlooks that I know we have much hope.

Stomping the Stigma

Along with Ashley, we hear from so many that they were shocked by their diagnosis, especially those who are younger and have never smoked a day in their lives—something we're hearing more and more.

"I didn't even think that lung cancer was a possibility for me, so it was very shocking. It was scary," Ashley told us in an interview. "At the time, my children were three and seven years old. I was just really scared, wondering if I would be here to raise my children. Would I be here to see them graduate high school and go to college, get married? All of those things that most people don't think about being a young mother. There were just a lot of questions swirling in my mind about my future."

Therefore, another aspect of hope in the lung cancer space is to ensure we stomp the stigma surrounding the disease. In a blog from Samantha Mixon, who was diagnosed with stage IV lung cancer at the age of thirty-three, she noted that the first question people asked following her diagnosis was, "Did you smoke?"

This was something that used to make her angry, until she realized it's what people are taught. "I know this question makes a lot of people angry. I used to get angry when asked—that is, until I came to realize that it's not the asker's fault," she said. "I would have asked the same thing before I actually got lung cancer. Society often teaches us that the only way you can get lung cancer is from smoking. This isn't true. There are so many contributing factors that people are unaware of, such as radon, air pollution, genetics, and just good old-fashioned bad luck."

As a community, we need to come together to stomp this stigma. Lung cancer affects individuals of all ages, sexes, and races. While we know how certain types can occur, there is still much more to learn. And it is the many patients and their loved ones sharing their stories that can help raise awareness: lung cancer is not just a smoker's disease.

Joining the Community

At first, Samantha also shared, she felt helpless when she received her diagnosis. And this is why I want to make sure everyone out there knows—you are not alone. You will never be alone on this journey.

"I've also made some incredible friends from all over the world through the lung cancer community," Samantha wrote. "We are united in a hunger and new appreciation for a life that most take for granted. Yes, I've lost many of those friends. And yes, it hurts when I do, but that's how I know I truly loved them and will see them again one day. No one can be replaced when they are a part of your heart.

"I see that we have this one life, one chance to make a difference in others and maybe make this world a better place. Evil didn't win. Cancer hasn't won and will never win, because I already have. I wouldn't take it back for a second. This is my life and this is my purpose—helping others."

One question I like to ask when wrapping up my interviews for articles, videos, or podcasts is: What would you say is your biggest piece of advice for a fellow patient? And now I ask myself the same question.

My reply? Get involved in the community.

It is with this community that we can continue to offer hope.

It is a great day to thrive. It is a great day to join a support group, advocate for yourself, or get involved with an advocacy group to continue to raise awareness surrounding lung cancer.

Together we can make a difference. Together we can offer hope— hope for the loved ones of those we've unfortunately lost to lung cancer. Hope for those affected today. Hope for tomorrow. And hope for many years to come.

For more information, go to curetoday.com

PREFACE

By Deborah Morosini, MD, MSW

My first reaction when Bonnie asked me to write this preface was: I won't ever be able to do that, maybe she should ask someone else. I don't know how I can say this to her politely, but that's what came up. Because the idea that I would ever be able to encapsulate what Bonnie means to me, and the impact she's had in my life, won't be effectively conveyed in the following passages. And so, I thought, maybe I should give up before I even begin. But that's not what Bonnie does. And so, that is not what I'm going to do either. With this caveat, here is my best effort at articulating how much Bonnie's mission and the community she has created resonates with my heart.

Bonnie Addario and her family parachuted into my life at a time of loss and it was her buoyancy, kindness, and activism that helped catalyze my own healing and philanthropic cancer activism. In 2006, I lost my sister, Dana Reeve, to lung cancer. Dana's life was one devoted to her family, the arts, and to helping others: in other words, to making the world a better place than she found it. She was nurturing, strong, funny, and inspiring, and my love for her has galvanized not only my own commitment to improving the lives of people with cancer, but has also cemented my friendship with Bonnie in whom I see these heartfelt qualities embodied and expressed.

I know nearly every person whose words fill these pages. Like them, I met Bonnie at a time when I was suffering acute personal loss, and trying to "keep it together" while raising two young sons, working at a Boston biotech startup, and mourning the loss of my sister, brother-in-law, and mother. But in that very moment of striving to keep everything together, I realized that, in the presence of Bonnie anyway, I didn't have to.

I felt an instant personal connection when we first met in San Francisco, at one of the early "Simply the Best" galas. Fred Marcus, her late and beloved oncologist was there, along with David Jablons, her skilled surgeon, and Melissa Lim, the pulmonologist who was instrumental in getting Bonnie to both of them. They were joined by Tony and "the girls," Andrea and Danielle. Another thing that became immediately apparent to me that night was Bonnie's mission: She didn't tell me this as much as I observed it and heard it from other people. She sought then, and seeks now, to embrace patients and their families and to shepherd them into a "new normal" with humor, grace, and support.

When Dana died, there was a paucity of research funding in lung cancer. Bonnie went where her strengths took her as a self-made success story, having risen to become president of the largest privately held oil company in the country. She leveraged her intelligence, charm, and persuasiveness to become the founder of Bonnie J. Addario Lung Cancer Foundation, and the Addario Lung Cancer Medical Institute (ALCMI). Much as the Christopher and Dana Reeve Foundation has a legacy of "care and cure," these two foundations—BJALCF and ALCMI—happily partnered to provide accessible, warm, welcome support for patients and their families alongside unique medical research in lung cancer and then merging it with the Lung Cancer Alliance to form the GO2 Foundation for Lung Cancer.

In the years since Dana died, incredible strides have been made in the treatment of lung cancer. Bonnie has been pivotal to moving many of these changes forward. With the advent of genomic testing and the rapid development of targeted therapies, patients have been enabled to achieve a better quality of life and longer survival times. Bonnie quickly grasped this connection and supported the cancer genomic testing movement fully. She gathered together a group of other lung cancer groups to support early efforts in genomic testing and Bonnie created the viral tagline: "Don't Guess – Test." The movement caught on, its message emblazoned across t-shirts and cute hoodies, and undoubtedly raised awareness and helped patients get testing.

Again, I was daunted to write this preface. The COVID-19 pandemic and the holidays fueled my procrastinations. Then I read this book you are about to read, and I'll confess I felt even MORE humbled by the honesty, the candor, and the bravery in the writing. Find a quiet spot, and enjoy. While it's a paradoxical recommendation, to "enjoy" a book about the experiences of people living with lung cancer, I urge you to let these stories, of humor, loss, fear, and the courage it takes to live a life richly imbued with all of these emotions at once, move you and change you, as they have changed me.

Thank you, Bonnie, for showing the way and, as always, lighting the way to a "living room."

Deborah Morosini, MD, MSW is a seasoned leader in cancer biopharma startups. She has two sons and lives in NYC. She is currently EVP / Chief of Clinical Affairs at Prelude Therapeutics.

INTRODUCTION

HOPE

They began arriving an hour before our scheduled start time, a number of them standing beneath the boldly stenciled letters that spell out H-O-P-E across the wall. It's the first thing they see when they open the door. On a crisp fall night in San Francisco in 2009, we have come together for a common purpose. There's an edge of nervous anxiety, nobody quite sure what to expect at our first gathering.

"Welcome to the Living Room," I greet everyone, introducing myself with a hug as attendees file past me, heading for a long table laden with appetizers, salads, bottled water, soda, and wine, all donated by local restaurants.

Most go for the wine. Those who've come straight from work are wearing suits or dresses; the ones who've come from home are dressed more casually. They all hold the same look in their eye that comes with gathering for a common purpose. They move tentatively, exchanging smiles and nods with total strangers with whom they share an indelible bond. People mill about introducing themselves, sharing stories of experiences everyone in the room can relate to all too well. The sound of their shoes on the shiny hardwood flooring is swallowed up by strategically placed carpets that add to a casual ambiance meant to replicate the comfort of home.

The lighting in the room is just right, warm and comfortable, in keeping with the welcoming atmosphere we'd sought to build. Plush sofas and conveniently placed coffee tables dominate the space, arranged to face a nesting of chairs set at the front of the room for all to see. That's where I'll be seated in a few minutes, right next to one of the world's foremost experts on lung cancer who'll be our first-ever guest speaker on this debut evening.

The majority of those coming through the door are lung cancer patients. Many are accompanied by family members or caregivers, while others are alone. They've all come for support, but this is no ordinary support group. Our plan, starting with this first night, is to bring in the foremost opinion leaders to speak about every facet of lung cancer, from diagnosis, screening, profiling, and treatment options to ongoing research and clinical trials. And our goal is to empower patients to become advocates themselves as a direct result of what they learn in the Living Room.

It's time to begin. My daughter stands up.

"Thank you all for coming. I'm Danielle, Bonnie's daughter. My mom is here with us tonight, thank God. She's right over there, and believe me, she's going to have a lot to say. But I'm here to welcome you. In the six years since lung cancer came into my life and turned my world upside down, the Living Room support and education group has been my dream!"

In that moment I see expressions change. What those gathered have long needed the most is about to be fulfilled. Perhaps it's the word "support" that makes people smile, that makes expressions go from just being there to listen to being present to find hope. The patients and survivors before me no longer feel like a gathering of individuals but more as a collective bonded by common hopes and dreams.

"I don't have an agenda for tonight," Danielle continues, "just a dream to create this place, this Living Room, where you can have a safe place to meet and talk about everything from high-level things like advanced genomic testing to eating mashed potatoes because the drugs you're taking are not letting you keep anything down. Maybe you're really mad at your doctor because he or she doesn't get back to you in a timely fashion, or maybe you're wondering when it's time to get a second opinion. Or perhaps you're dealing with family members or friends who have suddenly become absent because they just don't know how to deal with our *cancer*."

Danielle whispers that final word because for so long, especially with lung cancer, patients have been afraid of the stigma associated with it. Looking out at the audience, I can see the resistance to opening up breaking down. The burden of embarrassment and shame begins to melt away.

In the days following our first Living Room session, I heard from many attendees. "I left excited, so happy, and really appreciative that I found all of you," one patient wrote. "Thank you so much for the honesty, sharing your personal stories, all the advice and suggestions."

"I feel like I have a new 'family,'" another attendee said. "I look forward to seeing all of you again next month."

And with reactions like that, I knew we had made our Living Room open and welcoming, a place everyone who visits on the third Tuesday of every month could call home.

* * *

My own association with lung cancer actually predates my own diagnosis and treatment, but I didn't realize that until after my recovery. After my mother's death in 2005 to lung cancer we were going through her meager possessions that included four identical pairs of shoes in different colors she'd been wearing as long as I could remember when we came across a wooden box in which she kept her keepsakes and documents. One of those documents was her father's, my grandfather's, death certificate. We'd always thought he died of pneumonia, but according to the certificate, the cause was actually lung cancer, meaning the disease had left an indelible impression on my family long before I was even born.

After recovering from stage IIIB lung cancer and being declared cancer-free myself in 2006, I accepted an invitation to speak at a cancer support group in a major medical center nearby to where I live in Northern California. The experience was life-changing, not so much because of what was said but because of the setting itself.

Picture a large room with gray walls, gray carpeting, gray drapes, and gray folding chairs positioned around a gray oblong table—everything looked gray beneath the dull lighting. Even the people sitting there before me appeared gray. Nobody was living in that room. Instead of offering the support they'd come for, this place only reinforced the fact that they were dying. A support group setting should be a place where patients come to live, not die.

"How'd it go?" my husband, Tony, asked me when I got home that night.

"There was no hope in that room," I said.

And more than anything else, that's what these patients had come to this support group for. They wanted to believe they could beat this dreaded disease, and listening to people who had done precisely that should have been, quite literally, just what the doctor ordered. But this setting was a prescription for quite the opposite by tacitly confirming their worst fears. They came in seeking hope, but they sure didn't find it in that room.

Within days, I gathered my small team at the foundation that our family had started to advocate for lung cancer patients.

"We're going to start a support group," I announced. "And ours will be very different because it's going to be a place where people come to find hope, a room devoted to living, not dying."

That first standing-room-only night, over eighty guests walked into our Living Room through that door marked HOPE. For our first time out of the gate, that was certainly a formidable figure, but the modest success we achieved that night left me wishing we could reach more, far more.

"How do we reach more people, especially those who can't be here in person?" I asked my team. "It's not cost-effective to put a Living Room in every city. So how do we go to where the patients are?"

"Why don't we get a TV crew in here and we'll livestream it to the world," suggested Dani Gasparini, who did political interviews on TV in the San Francisco area.

"Let's do it!" I said, even though the technology to make it happen was way over my head.

The few cameras we placed in the room were unobtrusive and didn't stop anyone from wanting to share with those in the room, or with the more than a million people to date from 143 countries who've watched the live feed streamed on YouTube and Facebook Live. And if you miss a program, you can view it 24/7 on our website, where you also have access to our video library.

More often than not, when patients are in treatment, it's difficult for them to travel to or to attend an event at night, especially if they're working. Thanks to streaming, we've been able to bring the Living Room to them, right into homes like yours, where patients can relax and have a cup of tea or a glass of wine while they enjoy our company in a virtual realm.

When I went to Vienna in 2018 to speak at the annual International Association for the Study of Lung Cancer meeting, I spotted a beautiful young woman seated in the audience as I delivered my remarks from the podium. I could see from a distance the tears that streamed from her eyes. I made a mental note to go up to her to make sure she was okay and rushed over immediately after the session.

Before I could speak, she asked, "Can I get a hug?"

"Of course!"

"I have lung cancer," she said with an accent that I couldn't quite place.

We stepped away to a quieter area. She shared with me that she was from Australia.

"The day I was diagnosed," she said, her voice quivering, "I was terrified."

I hugged her again and held on to her longer.

"In Australia, there's no community support network," she explained. "I didn't know anyone I could lean on who understood what I was going through or could advise me on what to do. I felt alone. I searched the Web to look for some answers. That's when I found your Living Room."

"Wait, that had to be, what, three or four in the morning for you, right?"

"Yes. It was very early! I watched from under my covers in bed," she said, still holding back tears. "I saw other patients sharing their experiences. It gave me hope. I didn't feel alone anymore."

She cried. I cried. We hugged again for a long time.

Witnessing how the Living Room had helped her, I knew I'd found my path. I became convinced that my efforts might not only provide hope but also help reduce the number of individuals—a staggering million and a half people worldwide—who are diagnosed with lung cancer every year. That was my primary goal, and the Living Room helped me realize it by providing patients with knowledge that educated and empowered them to have intelligent, interactive discussions with their physicians.

After meeting this young woman in Vienna, I said to my team in California, "Let's make the Living Room interactive so patients don't just watch; they can chat live or email other patients or speakers in the room."

I love that today there are people in the chat room who've never met the people in the actual Living Room, but they nonetheless cheer them on through cyberspace with comments like, "Hey, tell so-and-so that I'm rooting for them."

One chat room participant from Prague said, "I've been watching your Living Room, and I see how you really believe in second opinions. I want to get a second opinion for my mum. Can you get me one?"

"Yes, of course," I said.

The next day, I called Dr. Fred Hirsch, the president of the International Association for the Study of Lung Cancer at the time.

"Fred, who have we got in Prague?"

I explained to him why I was asking, and he gave me the name of a doctor who had trained with him as a fellow.

"Here's his email address," he said.

I emailed the doctor:

YOU PROBABLY DON'T KNOW ME. I'M FROM THE UNITED STATES. I NEED A SECOND OPINION FOR A YOUNG WOMAN'S MOTHER IN PRAGUE.

"I know who you are from your Living Room," he wrote back. "Here's my cell phone. Give it to her, please, and I will take care of her mother."

The Living Room, after all, is where you come to live.

When I can't be at a Living Room session in person, I make sure to arrange my schedule to watch online so that I can listen to everyone. One of our sessions originated from a hospital in Florida. All the patients spoke Spanish, which was a first for our Living Room audience. I couldn't be there that night, so I watched it live on my laptop from my hotel room in Chicago. I didn't understand a word, but I took amazing pride in the fact that the Living Room was now multilingual and everyone was smiling, the universal language.

Lung cancer doesn't discriminate among race, creed, nationality, or socioeconomic levels, and, contrary to popular belief, the overwhelming majority of patients never smoked in their lives or gave it up years before their initial diagnosis. My overarching goal is to make lung cancer as survivable as any of the more common cancers like prostate, colon, or breast. In fact, lung cancer is the number-one cancer killer annually worldwide, taking more lives than those other three cancers combined. In 2020, nearly 150,000 people in the United States will die from lung cancer and nearly 225,000 Americans will be diagnosed, also more than the sum total of breast, colon, and prostate cancers. And yet, from a funding standpoint for research, lung cancer lags significantly behind those three cancers.

That needs to change.

* * *

By the time it was my turn to speak at our first Living Room on that December night in 2009, the room felt like one big family. Many new friendships had been made and many stories were shared, often for the first time in public. Our inaugural guests to the Living Room no longer felt hounded by the stigma of lung cancer and embarrassed by the shame. More than anything, they realized they weren't alone. We had given them and ourselves an early holiday gift, one that would be with all of us in the new year and beyond. I imagine that when many of them passed through the door at the end of the night, they took another look at the word over the entry way that had originally welcomed them:

HOPE

We are a nation of people who can do the impossible. We've always been able to defy the odds and achieve what the rest of the world never bothered to attempt. It's time to do that with lung cancer, which accounts for one-third of all cancer diagnoses. Think about that. If we can take down lung cancer, we're that much closer to eradicating cancer entirely. The treatment for so many other diseases and cancers has already been advanced by lung cancer research and targeted therapies that are now being applied with other patients. Genomics is leading the way in advanced medical research, and lung cancer is leading the way in genomics. One size doesn't fit all; not only is lung cancer teaching us that when it comes to treatment, it's also teaching us how to precisely tailor a program for an individual patient. And thanks in large part to lung cancer research, we will see that applied to a myriad of other illnesses, cancer and otherwise.

So much of the past year has been about the rise of the Black Lives Matter movement, in large part because of the murder of George Floyd in Minneapolis at the hands, and feet, of police. Remember George Floyd's final words?

I can't breathe.

Well, that's also how lung cancer patients feel. They can't breathe either. Since president Richard Nixon declared war on cancer in 1971, we have lost at least forty million people to lung cancer. The injustice of that is staggering, and we're not going to lose forty million more. We can't let that happen, and that's why I'm writing this book. It's for my children and grandchildren and all the people I have met on my own journey, to save their lives. The injustice has to stop too.

Since our first night in San Francisco back in 2009, nearly a million and a half people have visited the Living Room, either in person or in the virtual sense. But we want to reach more, we want to do more to get the message of hope out there. So we created this book, in the pages of which you're going to meet lung cancer patients and survivors, heroes all, who've found a way not only to live with lung cancer but to thrive as they fight to overcome the obstacles the disease plants before their plans and the setbacks it imposes on their dreams. Lung cancer gives no quarter and takes no prisoners. But neither do these brave men and women who, armed with the latest weapons modern medicine has to offer, have no intention of giving up the fight. They are our guests in this literary Living Room.

This is what lung cancer looks like. The people you are about to meet are its face. They are you, they are me, they are all of us.

But this isn't really a book about lung cancer. It's a book about people with terminal diseases who find the courage to live and thrive. They want to see their children graduate from high school, then college, perhaps marry and start families of their own. They want to become grandparents and grow old with their loved ones, to see everything they should be able to see.

I'm so fortunate because I survived, one of the 17 percent or so who do, and I'm even more fortunate for having the chance to meet all the people you're about to meet in these pages. They are my new heroes, the very definition of what it means to be brave. They don't give in and they don't give up, men and women who come to the Living Room hopeless and leave hopeful.

So come right in. Join us and make yourself comfortable. Our session is about to begin.

FROM MY DAUGHTER ANDREA...

My sister, Danielle, and I were opening a boutique at the time my mom was diagnosed. She waited until the very day we opened to tell us because she knew we would have abandoned all our plans if she'd told us before, and she didn't want that. It was a horrible time in my life for the simple fact that losing my mom was not an option. And that was exacerbated by the fact that none of us knew anything about lung cancer. So we rolled up our sleeves and decided as a family we would become part of the decision-making process. We would be with her all the time, going to her appointments and being there for her through all of her treatments. We'd always been close. When my mom and dad separated, my sister and brother and my mom and I became the "Four Musketeers," to the point that whenever one of us went out, we wouldn't just say "Bye," we'd also say "I love you."

My mom quickly realized that if she could be diagnosed with lung cancer, anybody could be diagnosed with lung cancer. I know that angered her, and she turned her attention to what she could do to change it, along with how the disease was treated and perceived. Sixteen years later, I don't think she realizes the impact she's made on so many people. As a family I know that we have a share in making that impact, and I know she takes great pride in that. But I want to make sure she's enjoying her own life too, enjoying every minute she has with the family she's created. I want her to have the same impact on my kids she has had with me.

Recently there was a family in our foundation offices that reminded me so much of us sixteen years ago. A brother and a sister asking questions they desperately needed answers for. It was very emotional, and it reminded me of how important it was going to be for them to stick together the way we did and support each other when they're having a bad day, just like we did. I think knowing we were so close, that we were in this together, made my mom fight the disease even harder because she didn't want to miss out on her future with us and her grandchildren. Having 100 percent family support gave her one less thing to worry about, so she could focus on getting better herself. No one can go through a fight like that alone. That's what we preach at the foundation. And if you don't have that kind of support around you, we'll find a way to get it for you, thanks to my mom, her vision.

People take so much for granted, including the kind of family bond they have. I have friends who don't talk to their siblings or maybe even their parents. I don't understand that, how they can live that way, and how they'd deal with something like lung cancer if it came their way. I remember when I was a kid how my friends thought it was weird that we always said "I love you" to each other. They didn't get it, didn't get that we did it because we never knew if that might be the last time we saw that person again.

If I had one wish, it would be that my mom was never diagnosed with lung cancer, that nobody ever got diagnosed with lung cancer. But my second wish would be that she would stop once in a while and smell the roses of all the great things she's done. I'd love to have her enjoy the rest of her life, but I know if she heard me say that, she'd tell me she *is* enjoying her life, because helping others is what she enjoys more than anything.

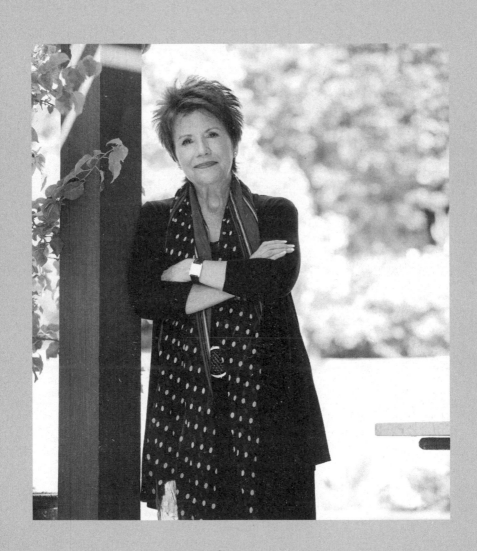

PROLOGUE

My Story: Diagnosis

A nagging pain shot across the left side of my chest in late 2003, constant but not agonizing. It had appeared and disappeared for almost a year, along with a chronic, though mild, cough.

I was never good at going to doctors. Even when I had pneumonia, I only went reluctantly after work to one of those urgent care centers for treatment. So I ignored the chest pains and cough, until the day my husband, Tony, and I were at the Laguna Seca Raceway in Monterey, California, for a work-related visit. I couldn't catch a breath and could barely walk across the infield or climb the steps without stopping. I thought I was going to collapse.

Tony grabbed hold of me. "What's the matter?"

"This 'thing' in my chest is really bothering me today," I panted. "I can't breathe."

"Okay, that's it," he said. "You're going to the doctor. Now."

My primary physician sent me for a barrage of tests, including an echocardiogram. He was sure the pain was related to my heart. But the

1

tests came back normal. So they ordered more tests. I saw a bevy of specialists, who suspected everything from bronchitis to a slipped disk.

"No, I've got chest pains," I insisted.

My primary ordered physical therapy anyway. My predicament was not unusual at all in the annuls of lung cancer, a notoriously difficult disease to diagnose because the symptoms suggest so many possibilities. For that reason, they failed to order a CT scan that could have detected the kind of telltale tumors that can hide behind the heart and ribs.

One neurologist finally diagnosed the symptoms as coming from a herniated disk in my neck. I bought into his theory and started taking Vioxx—an anti-inflammatory drug—to dull the pain. It reduced the pressure on my chest, but just when I'd gotten used to taking it every day, a study came out that showed Vioxx could induce a heart attack or increase stroke risk in some users, so it was pulled off the market. My pain quickly came raging back. After a cardiologist took chest X-rays that also came back normal, I decided I'd have to learn to live with the pain. What choice did I have?

Tony was less accepting than I. He embarked on a mission to get to the bottom of whatever was happening to my body. He found a newspaper article about an independent center that did full-body scans that could detect early signs of cancer and heart disease.

"Let's get you in there," he said. "I'll get one too. What have we got to lose?"

Full-body scans weren't reimbursable services and generally required a doctor's referral. We didn't have one, but we explored our options anyway. The closest facility, in San Jose, California, had a long waiting list for the procedure.

Tony was like a caged tiger, ready to go out and buy a machine himself if he had to. Then space opened up, and we paid nearly $2,000 each to have the scans done.

The results came back quickly.

"You're fine, Tony," the radiologist said.

Then he turned to me. "See this right here, Bonnie?" he asked, scan in hand.

A shadow covered a part of my left lung and aorta.

"You need to take this to your primary care physician, today," the radiologist said, a grave edge to his voice that made me feel as if I'd swallowed ground glass.

I nodded and called immediately for an appointment. Those few steps into my primary's office the next day felt like the longest walk I'd ever taken. Managing my breathing was easy, given that I was unconsciously holding my breath.

"Bonnie," he said. "You have a growth, and it looks suspicious."

"Suspicious? As in *cancer*?"

I could barely bring myself to say the word, although by this time I couldn't help but consider it. The CT scan had revealed something all the other tests missed. Still, given the absence of a definitive finding or diagnosis, my doctor ordered a follow-up CT scan to provide a more detailed picture and determine the size and exact location of the tumor.

"Get it done right away," he urged. "If I get the results tomorrow, I'll call you. Otherwise, I'll check up on you after I return from my vacation next week."

Talk about feeling powerless. And exactly one week later, my phone rang at 7:00 a.m. Never a good thing.

"I need you to come in and meet with our pulmonologist," my primary care doctor stated.

"Not good news?"

"No. Your scan doesn't look good."

A cold wave swept down my body. My hand shook so hard that it took three tries to hang up the phone. I was fifty-five years old, president of one of the largest privately held oil companies in the US after starting work there fifteen years before. I was used to fighting for everything I achieved, to being in control. But I had the terrifying feeling this was going to be something I couldn't control and might not be able to successfully fight.

Tony was out of town, but I couldn't bear to be alone. So I called my oldest daughter, Danielle, who had long shown deep interest in the medical world and I knew could offer comfort as well as knowledge.

"Can you come over?"

"Sure. Everything okay?"

"Just come on over. I need you."

When she arrived, I poured both of us a glass of wine.

Danielle looked at me doing that before the workday even started, her face paling. "What's going on, Mom?"

I took as deep a breath as I could. "We don't have definitive results from the tests yet," I said, trying to keep my voice steady, "but they saw something in the scans."

"What does that mean?"

How do I say this? "There's a tumor on my lung and aorta."

Danielle's eyes widened. Her face got paler.

"Don't tell your brother or sister!" I pleaded. "Not yet, anyway. Let me find out what's going on for sure first."

Tears formed at the corners of Danielle's eyes. I looked away from her to prevent my own tears from falling. Then I grabbed her hands.

"Everything's going to be fine," I said. "I'm not going to worry about this, and I don't want you to stress. Let's just take this one day at a time."

While most people were now beginning their workdays, we finished the bottle of wine in silence. And after Danielle left, I gave myself a good talking to, telling myself that worrying about the future only invites anxiety.

When Tony came home, we met with the pulmonologist who'd already reviewed the films and proceeded to poke around me for what seemed like hours.

"You have a tumor," he confirmed. "And it's in a precarious place."

I took a deep breath and let the words sink in, holding back the urge to speak. He held up my new scan to show how the tumor was on my aorta and subclavian artery. Every time my heart beat, the tumor beat with it. That's what was causing my dull, constant pain.

"So, do I have cancer? Do I have *lung cancer*?"

"Well, we're going to have to get a biopsy to see what kind of cancer it is."

I felt numb. I've never done "being vulnerable" well. I never allowed myself to cry in front of people. If I have to cry, which is rare, I do it in the shower. I took a long shower that day.

Danielle and my other daughter, Andrea, were about two weeks away from opening a little boutique nearby in downtown San Carlos. I walked through the back alley of their store the next day and asked them to join me outside.

"I may have lung cancer."

Just like that, I came out and said it, and silence filled the air between us. We were all speechless.

"We're not opening the store," Danielle and Andrea insisted.

"You absolutely are! If I can be strong and move forward, you can too. We can't give in to this!"

Due to the tumor's location, we had a tough time finding someone who would agree to perform the required biopsy. My first biopsy was scheduled at a community hospital, the kind of facility that often doesn't have the same standard of care as a major academic center for lung cancer. A staff member escorted Tony and me into a small room about the size of a broom closet. File cabinets and storage boxes were everywhere. The only resemblance to an operating room was the examination table. Not exactly a recipe to inspire confidence.

Getting to my tumor, which was located dangerously close to my heart, wasn't easy. The "procedure" began with the doctors using two Q-tip-like chopsticks, each about six feet long. They put cocaine on the edges and shoved them up my nostrils to deaden my senses and nerves. The lead doctor then pushed them up higher and higher until they were going down the back of my throat. That's how he anesthetized me. Then he snaked a tiny camera up my nose and down into my lungs to where they thought the tumor was.

The whole agonizing process seemed almost barbaric. Because the tumor was lying on my aorta and he was afraid of doing damage there, the doctor eventually conceded defeat and came up empty.

"We'll have to have a surgeon go in there and see what's going on. Exploratory surgery is the only way we're going to see what's happening."

But that turned out not to be an option for me. In fact, I didn't seem to have any options at all.

* * *

With Christmas just a few weeks away, I sat in my kitchen one afternoon reading a newspaper, and came across a small article I could have easily missed but thankfully didn't.

"Oh my God!" I leaped up from the kitchen chair, flashing page ten of the *San Mateo County Times*. "Look at this," I said to Tony, holding the paper up so he could read a headline:

SEQUOIA HOSPITAL TESTS LUNG-CANCER PROGRAM

He put aside the dish he'd learned to make in his post-retirement cooking classes and moved in closer to read the brief article with me.

"For the past several months, a University of California San Francisco (UCSF) surgeon has been coming to the hospital once a week to treat difficult lung cancer cases that would generally be referred to the University. 'We're testing the water but the goal is to make it a permanent thing,' said Dr. David Jablons, chief thoracic surgeon to the University."

"I have to see Dr. Jablons!" I proclaimed, ready to jump into the car in that very second.

* * *

I had no problem going for a second opinion. Even today, I stress with newly diagnosed lung cancer patients the importance of getting one. I meet a lot of "Bonnies" out there, terrified by the horrible diagnosis they just received. They're paralyzed. They don't know how to make the next decision on their care. I urge them to do what I did: look for better physicians and better therapies. I tell them, "You need a second opinion."

It's tough enough having lung cancer before we even get to the part about how people look at you when they find out. As I did initially, they fall prey to the common mythology that lung cancer is a smoker's cancer. It's not. Around 60 percent of newly diagnosed people either never smoked or quit smoking decades ago. People look at you and figure you brought it on yourself, that you don't deserve to live. As Barbara Denson, a lung cancer patient who succumbed to the disease in 2013, said shortly before her death, "I never smoked, but smoking is going to kill me."

Since President Nixon declared war on cancer in 1971, forty million people have been lost to lung cancer alone. The bubonic plague, a.k.a. the Black Death, killed twenty-five million. The Spanish flu outbreak of 1918 allegedly took as many as fifty million lives (most estimates put the number at significantly less than that, closer to twenty million). And those are considered to be among the major pandemics in human history, even though neither killed as many as lung cancer has.

Look at it another way. Every day we lose 450 people in the United States alone to lung cancer—that's every single day. Now imagine waking up this morning to the news that the same number died in the crash of a jumbo jet. Sad and terrible, yes, but quickly forgotten; that is until you wake up the next morning to another jumbo jet crashing and 450 more lives lost. Same thing the third morning. Imagine the desperation and resolve to do something about it, to stop it from happening again. My point is that lung cancer is like a jumbo jet crashing every single day, but where is the concurrent desperation and resolve?

Life feels over when you get any cancer diagnosis, but lung cancer is especially nefarious given that people are as likely to shake their heads at you as shake your hand warmly and wish you good luck. After all, you brought it on yourself, right? We had a visitor to the Living Room once who told people she had breast cancer instead of lung cancer so she wouldn't be frowned upon. As the saying goes, breast cancer patients get casseroles while lung cancer patients get stigmatized.

I couldn't accept that. Since you've joined me today in our literary Living Room, you know I'm one of the lucky ones. And that puts me in the unique position to advocate for those who are following my path, hopefully to recovery. Surviving lung cancer was like being granted a second chance, and I intend to do everything with it I can, starting with educating both the public and lung cancer patients on the realities of the disease. That it's a disease suffered by young people as well as older ones, and that no one should have to bear the additional burden of being stigmatized

To that point, one of the major efforts I've taken on of late has been to initiate a medical trial called the Genomics of Young Lung Cancer to determine why so many young never-smokers, who are fit and active, with their whole lives in front of them, are being diagnosed with the disease. No matter your age, whether you're twenty-five or eighty-five, lung cancer is like a scarlet letter on your forehead. My mission in life became to see that stigma erased so that patients need not feel like second-class citizens. Feeling ashamed was not acceptable to me.

First, though, I had to get better myself.

* * *

Sequoia Hospital is a visionary community hospital that's known worldwide. Tony and I had become donors after one of the hospital's cardiac physicians took wonderful care of my dad. I'd even joined their foundation board. I was president of my second company at that time, and such appointments were considered kind of routine for those holding such a position.

Not anymore in my case.

I called the board president and explained to her what was going on with me and how urgent it was to get my treatment moving.

"I'll get in touch with Dr. Melissa Lim," she offered. "She's the pulmonologist who worked with Dr. Jablons in his UCSF lab and helped to start the lung cancer program here."

Barely an hour later, my phone rang.

"Bonnie, go get your scans from the other hospital network," Dr. Lim instructed. "Bring them to me first thing tomorrow."

She was waiting when I arrived the next morning and reviewed them on the spot. "Now give me forty-eight hours," she said, without further comment.

Dr. Lim used that time to reach out to the major academic hospitals in the area to get their opinions on possible courses of treatment.

"It's inoperable," said one.

"It's too dangerous to perform surgery," from a second.

The third response was altogether different.

"I took your scans over to UCSF," Dr. Lim said. "Dr. Jablons wants to see you right away."

I sat in the waiting room of another physician, oncologist Dr. Fred Marcus, the next day, nervous but allowing myself a modicum of hope. I'd become good at handling life's crises on my own, but that day I was glad to have Tony and the kids with me. With multiple sets of ears, we wouldn't miss any information, good or bad. We were all a bit jittery but sat there quietly. Tony clutched my hand the entire time; Danielle and Andrea never moved more than a yard from me.

The doors sprang open, and a young man rushed through. Our eyes followed him as he whisked past the receptionist to exit through another door that led to the examination rooms.

Maybe that runner has my scans, I thought.

Moments later, a nurse escorted the four of us into a small, sterile examination room cluttered with a few chairs.

"This is Dr. Fred Marcus," she said, pointing to the seasoned oncologist. "And this is your thoracic surgeon, Dr. David Jablons."

My mouth dropped—Dr. Jablons was the young man I'd seen charging down the hallway.

"That was you?" I said to him, pointing toward the waiting room. "Are you even old enough to drive to the hospital?"

"Thanks, but I'm fifty."

After the formalities, Dr. Jablons motioned for Tony and me to sit. He folded his arms, holding my charts close to his chest. With my eyes locked on his face, I searched for a clue of what was to come, but his expression was blank, giving nothing away.

"Your lung cancer is stage IIIB," he said, cutting to the chase. "You have the equivalent of localized early stage cancer."

I squeezed Tony's hand. Speechless, I just stared.

"It's not biologically aggressive," he continued, "but because it's invading your aorta, it's staged as IIIB…"

I sank deeper into my chair.

"Fortunately, though, it hasn't metastasized yet to any other organs." I exhaled.

"It's fortunate that you recognized something was wrong early on and were financially able to pay for the full-body scans. Another four or five weeks, we might not have been able to do anything."

"So, you can do *something*?" I managed, my voice shaky.

"Here's what I recommend." He pulled a pen out of his pocket and started drawing on the white paper stretched across the examination table. "This is your heart. This is where we can do this…and that…and that…I'll just take it out and then…"

I don't remember all of his words as he described the tumor's encroachment in the aorta's space. I do remember, though, that in terms of operative mortality, on a scale of one to ten, with ten being ridiculous, he rated me somewhere around a nine-point-five.

Dr. Jablons drew out everything on that paper so I could understand his team's proposed plan—where the problem was and all the technical issues involved. He wanted me entirely invested in the whole process. Then he ripped the paper off the exam table and pinned it to the wall like it was a Matisse. And to this man whose creative tool was a scalpel instead of a brush, that's exactly what it was. To me, it looked like senseless scribblings, but I hung on to his every word.

"Fred and I agreed that we're going to start you on some pretty nasty chemotherapy every Friday and do radiation every Monday, Tuesday, Wednesday, Thursday, and Friday for about nine rounds."

My throat closed.

Receiving the diagnosis of a potentially terminal disease, be it cancer or something else, is a full body blow. I'd already braced myself for that, but listening to Dr. Jablons lay out the rigors of the treatment protocol hit me even harder.

"If we can shrink this tumor just enough to safely peel it off your heart and aorta," Dr. Jablons continued, "we'll be able to look at surgery."

With my eyes still fixed on his drawings, I asked what any business executive would: "What's plan B?"

The doctors exchanged looks.

"Bonnie, there is no plan B," Dr. Jablons stated plainly.

I was incredulous. *"No plan B?"*

"Look, if you don't do plan A, the tumor will crush your aorta, and you will bleed to death."

My head dropped down toward my chest.

"You have to have this surgery," Dr. Jablons said.

I couldn't look at the girls or Tony. I'd dreaded that moment. No more tests, biopsies, or second opinions. I faced a fate I couldn't fix. I couldn't make it go away or control the outcome. Accepting that reality was tougher than accepting the diagnosis. I slipped deep into a meditative kind of thought where I felt detached, as if I weren't really there.

"Bonnie?" Dr. Jablons said. "Bonnie, this is serious, difficult, and dangerous. But that's what I do."

I looked at him straight in the eye, inspired by his confidence. "You're the guy."

"Can we go ahead and schedule you for the chemo and radiation?"

I heard myself speak like it was someone else doing the talking. "Yes. Let's do this."

I knew so little then about lung cancer, even though I'd lost four relatives to the disease, three of whom were stage IV (the most advanced), including my mother and maternal grandfather, who we initially thought had died from pneumonia until we found that death certificate years later.

Tony, the kids, and I practically lived on the internet and in libraries searching deeper for as much information as we could find about lung cancer. What little we found was dire and hopeless, and there was practically no information at all on how to live with the disease. Also appalling was the lack of support groups for lung cancer patients and their loved ones. There was no place to go to share experiences or just ask questions.

Sequoia Hospital was just blocks away from our house, which meant I didn't have to drive all the way to San Francisco every day to receive my chemo and radiation treatments. That was something anyway, and as with everything else, Tony and the kids were right there with me every day, no matter how much I told them they didn't have to be.

The double dose of chemo was painful and draining. It quickly killed everything: my hair, nails, eyebrows, and appetite. I lost weight and felt weak all the time. Tony would offer to make me one of his fabulous gourmet meals, but all I could eat was Jell-O and cranberry juice, which was still plenty more than many patients can.

I didn't want to be a burden to Tony and the kids, so I tried to keep to myself as much as I could during the treatments.

"Let them in," the radiation nurse advised. "It helps them cope as much as it helps you."

That was hard advice for me to take since, thanks to my nature, I was used to being in charge and doing things for myself. And besides that, I felt guilty. Tony had just entered retirement, but instead of filling his days doing things that gave him the most joy, he filled them accompanying me to all my appointments, providing updates on my condition to family and friends, and making decisions I couldn't, wouldn't, or shouldn't make myself. I let him in a little at a time, still trying to do way too much for myself.

One day when I couldn't make it to the bathroom to throw up, Tony found me cleaning up after myself. He finished the cleanup process and helped me into bed.

"I told you before—you have to let me help you get through this."

That was the day I let him in. I loved that he talked to me like I was his wife, not as so many others did, which was like a patient.

A couple of weeks into the chemo and radiation treatments, I told Tony I wanted the whole family to spend the weekend at our Lake Tahoe, Nevada, vacation home, where we went every year around the same time. I didn't know when—or if—I'd make it back there again.

Tahoe was cold and alluring, a winter wonderland with glistening white powder covering the mountaintops, beautiful sunsets, and a crisp chill in the air. Just as the snow fell from the sky, my hair fell from my head in clumps. The girls and I went wig shopping. In fact, I bought dozens of wigs in different styles. I generally wore my hair long, but I figured I'd be adventurous and go with a bob. I tried it on before dinner one night and then tore it off.

"I'll never wear this again," I said, staring at myself in the mirror. "Girls, it's horrible!"

Nothing made me more aware of having cancer than feeling that thing on my head. We grabbed an electric razor.

"Let's just get this over with," I said. "I'm done. Let's do this."

We had a shaving party in my bedroom. The girls brought in two bottles of champagne and orange juice, and we made mimosas while Danielle shaved off my tresses. She and Andrea even made little lines and funny curvy things on my head. We laughed until there was no champagne—or hair—left.

From then on, I wore biker do-rags. I had them in different colors. I did my best not to change my routine. And since the girls went ahead and opened their boutique, I visited it as often as I could, wearing my beanies and buying things I didn't need.

Thankfully, the full-court press of gruesome chemo and radiation treatments had done its job, but my tumor was still in a dicey spot: on top of my heart and invading my aorta. But it had shrunk enough to let Dr. Jablons do what he'd described in our initial meeting amid all those drawings.

I was finally cleared for surgery.

You're about to meet Gina Hollenbeck, who has a wonderful and heart-felt story to tell that highlights, among other things, the vital importance of caregivers and the effects of the disease on family members as well. That makes this an opportune time to share how life changes for the friends and loved ones of a lung cancer patient. The following is excerpted from an article in CURE *magazine by Dara Chadwick in May 2019 and is reprinted with permission.*

Relationships, including the roles and responsibilities of each person, often come under a microscope following a cancer diagnosis. "The dynamics that already existed in the partnership set the tone for what happens next," says Sarah Paul, MSW, a licensed clinical social worker and child, adolescent, and young adult program manager at CancerCare in New York City, a national organization providing free professional support services to those affected by cancer. For some men, taking on new roles in the relationship poses an additional challenge, on top of their partner having cancer, she says.

These new duties might include acting as a patient advocate, which requires organization, talking with medical professionals, and managing the details of treatment. Some men become information managers, responsible for updating friends and family on their partner's status. Other men may step into the role of primary parent for the first time—a particular challenge when Mom has been the main caretaker and children might not be used to listening to Dad, Paul says. "Some dads say things like 'I'm not a good parent' when they feel like the kids aren't listening to them."

The changes can be tough on women too, especially if their relationship tended toward a more traditional gender split of roles. "Little things she did may fall to the wayside," Paul says. "It can be overwhelming if you're not prepared for it." Still, such role reversals aren't always negative. "There's often an opportunity to learn more about your partner and strengthen your relationship," she says.

Finding support is key to managing the physical, emotional, and practical stresses for men in the caregiver role, especially because men tend to experience the role in more isolation, says Allison Applebaum, PhD, a licensed clinical psychologist and director of the Caregivers Clinic at Memorial Sloan Kettering Cancer Center in New York City. Some men are self-isolating, saying things like "I feel alone in this role," she says, adding that others struggle to find a support network because there are fewer men in the caregiver role.

Caregivers also need support for the practical challenges they face. Men who manage transporting their partner to treatment and medical appointments and providing care at home may require help with taking care of young children or chauffeuring older kids to sports and other activities. They may also need to ask for time off work to care for their partner, which can create financial stress or job uncertainty. To find support, they may need to ask for help—something that isn't always easy to do, Paul says.

Applebaum, who has written a new book, *Cancer Caregivers*, says men may also benefit from a caregiver mentoring program, an informal support system that pairs experienced and new caregivers. Comprehensive cancer centers and organizations, such as the American Cancer Society, can help caregivers connect with resources and support groups. "Sometimes, just one conversation is all it takes," she says. "Some people just want information. It's about finding the right type of support for you. Sometimes people say, 'I'm not the patient, so why do my feelings matter?' But in a family, you're all affected."

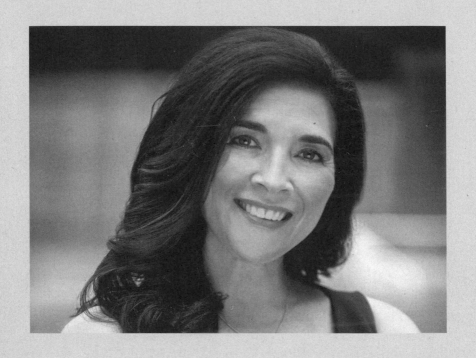

1

Gina Hollenbeck

There's a photograph accompanying a profile of Gina Hollenbeck picturing her smiling up from a hospital bed, fist-pumping with her beloved husband, Greg. Not yet forty, the nonsmoking, healthy mother of two boys had been suffering a stubborn, persistent cough and weight loss for months when she finally decided to get a chest X-ray. A nurse herself, Gina called a friend at an imaging lab to schedule an appointment.

"Just get an order for one from your doctor," the friend advised.

"How much does it cost?" Gina asked, fearful of delaying the process any further.

"Seventy-five dollars."

"Never mind the order," Gina said. "I'll pay for it myself."

Needing an answer for what had been ailing her, she discussed her symptoms during a routine office visit with her OB-GYN, who thought her symptoms might be the result of seasonal allergies. When two weeks on Zyrtec produced no improvement in her symptoms, and her cough continued to worsen, she decided on probing her condition further with that chest X-ray at a nearby Memphis, Tennessee, hospital, which a technician read right away.

"There's something going on here I don't like," he told her. "You need to go see a pulmonologist."

"When?"

"Now, as in today."

When the pulmonologist recommended to her couldn't see Gina as a new patient for two months, she was advised to go to the emergency room. She had, after all, been sensing something was wrong for some months now, and the signs were only getting stronger.

"So I walked into the ER with the chest X-ray under my arm, looking young and healthy, and told the receptionist that I was a nurse and knew I didn't look sick but I thought there might be something seriously wrong with me. Fortunately, they took me seriously and scheduled me for a CT scan right away."

That scan showed a number of tumors, though the initial thinking of the doctors was that they weren't cancer.

"They noted my persistent cough and the fact that I'd lost a little weight. But how could a thirty-eight-year-old woman, who never smoked and had just run a 5K, have lung cancer? They sent me to see a pulmonologist, who asked me to come back the next day for a biopsy. He took sections of a tumor, and I asked him the obvious question: 'Do you think it's cancer?'"

Gina tells me that he actually didn't, believing it was either a fungus or pneumonia. He needed to find out which so he could figure out how to treat her. But that didn't make sense to Gina, and sure enough, the lab results confirmed tumor cells were present. Only then did he say, "It's cancer."

I don't know Gina well, but after she enthusiastically agreed to be interviewed for this story and we spoke on the phone, I feel like I've known her forever.

As Gina and I talk, I find myself looking at that picture of her smiling up from her hospital bed. It's morning where I am in the Bay Area, early afternoon back east in Memphis. There's an ease to Gina's conversational tone, as if she's adept at making people comfortable in her presence, even if that presence is three thousand miles away and strictly via voice. This call is about her, but she wants to talk about me and my experiences just as much. So here we are, women from two different generations who share the common bond of lung cancer.

To prepare for our conversation, I watched a number of videos in which Gina is featured. Several were filmed at the NFL Experience for a promotion coordinated by the Chris Draft Family Foundation. There was Gina on camera, bursting with life, energy, and hope. Her enthusiasm explodes off the screen, exuding the magnetism and charisma of a rock star.

"I'm Gina Hollenbeck," she says, standing next to her husband and caregiver, Greg, "and we're here to tackle lung cancer together, because it takes a team to fight lung cancer."

The short video ends with Gina laying waste to a tackling dummy the same way she's attacked her lung cancer and pounded it straight into the turf.

"I have two young sons," an equally buoyant Gina says, after introducing herself as a speaker at the National Lung Cancer Roundtable, "and I have a husband who loves me very, very much, and I have stage IV lung cancer."

She wants the audience to know about her family first and foremost, all she stands to lose if that tackling dummy starts fighting back again. That's her priority, her motivation, and inspiration to stay ahead of a dreaded adversary that doesn't respect the kind of boundaries that enclose a football field. Lung cancer may be relentless in stealing life, but you get the sense Gina is equally relentless in holding on to hers.

"I want you to know why I'm so passionate about advocating for lung cancer," she continues in her speech, going on to detail her life prior to her diagnosis. The regimens she went through to take care of herself, the utter incredulity over the fact that she could contract the disease in the first place. Everyone she saw initially agreed on one thing and one thing only: whatever you've got, it's not lung cancer.

The doctors were right, until they were proved to be wrong. And when they told Gina initially there was nothing they could do, she refused to accept that prognosis. She knew they could do better than that, and if they couldn't, she'd find someone who could. She had too much to live for to accept anything less.

As a nurse, Gina was no stranger to sickness. When it came to herself, though, that experience provided little comfort. And her case is emblematic of the attitude that best defines lung cancer patients who ultimately gain successful outcomes: instead of asking, "Why me?" Gina chose to adopt a different approach: "Why *not* me?"

"I knew as a health care worker," she says, "that I could beat this, that I *would* beat this. I'm going to find the right doctors here in Memphis, the best care. I was going to win."

Gina threw herself into the fight instead of retreating to the corner and absorbing blow after blow. She had a family, after all, and needed to be strong for them as well as herself.

"It never occurred to me I might lose, not for one minute."

As dreaded as her diagnosis was, it came only through Gina's personal persistence, knowledge of her own body, and confidence in her belief that something was wrong. Her case serves as an example of the kind of empowerment that has come to increasingly define those patients with successful outcomes—patients who do their own legwork, their own research into the latest therapies, and refuse to take no for an answer when it comes to both diagnosis and treatment.

"I was diagnosed on October 27, 2015," Gina recalls, the date memorialized in part because of the family's annual Halloween party that was fast approaching. "And I decided I wasn't going to tell anyone at the party that I'd just been given ten months to live. How do you tell somebody something like that? I didn't want the party to be about cancer. If this was going to be the last time we had this party, I wanted everyone to have a good time. Greg and I were really adamant about keeping my diagnosis a secret. When we started telling people a few days later, nobody could believe a person who, outwardly anyway, was the picture of health could be that sick. Every time I told somebody else, I felt like I was receiving the diagnosis, that death sentence, all over again, and it was hard to put the people I was closest to and loved the most in the world through that. I felt I was hurting them.

"Their response floored me. The whole community rallied around me. They started a Facebook page called Gina's Army so people could offer messages of support and encouragement. Whenever I got really, really down, Gina's Army would be right there. Even the kids at my oldest son's school got involved. You know, before I got cancer the world always seemed like this big, bad place. Getting sick allowed me to see how kind people are, doing things they didn't have to do. Loving, giving, supporting. I came to see the world as a wonderful place, and sometimes it takes facing the kind of adversity I was facing to see that. All that support helped me accept the fact there was a good chance I could die. But so can anybody, at pretty much anytime—you just never know. So I really had no reason to be afraid to die. I decided to focus on living instead. I'd been given this day today, so why don't I work to get the most out of it? Same thing with tomorrow and the next day, if I'm lucky enough to get those too. Getting the chance to live made me more aware of living, paying attention and being thankful for every little thing. I don't have the same anger, the same stress, because now I know every day might be my last. I'm not guaranteed tomorrow; no one is. So why not make the most of today?"

More than four years after her initial diagnosis, Gina looks and feels great. Her energy and verve are so demonstrative that I feel like she's sitting in the room with me instead of being three thousand miles away. I don't know how long we've been talking, but I don't want our call to end. I want to hold on to Gina because of everything she represents. And I'm afraid of what might happen if I let her go, because the harsh realities of cancer haven't gone away.

There are four targeted therapies generally prescribed for the ALK-positive lung cancer she's suffering from. The first three all worked for a time, before the cancer grew smart enough to outwit them in each case. The growing resistance of tumor cells to one treatment after another is exceedingly common for lung cancer patients. Gina's now in the middle of the fourth treatment. The last one.

"But that's only today," she says with unbridled optimism that continues to burst through the phone line. "If and when this treatment stops working, there might be three more available, with others coming down the pipe. In the four years since I was diagnosed, we've already come so far. Back then insurance didn't cover bio-testing for targeted markers because they were considered experimental. Now they're FDA approved. I was diagnosed and then treated for lung cancer, and I've never actually felt sick, and right now I've never felt better in my life. It used to be there was a step approach to lung cancer treatment. You start with one drug, progress to another, and so on. But you don't have to do that anymore. You can skip steps and proceed straight to the treatment most likely to produce positive results in your case. So I'm not thinking ten years down the road, I'm thinking one. One year, one day at a time."

Numbers don't lie, but neither in Gina's case do they tell the whole story.

"It wasn't just me who got cancer," she recalls, "it was our whole family. 'We got cancer' was the way we'd all describe it. My husband, Greg, was with me every step of the way. He's a pilot for FedEx with no medical knowledge whatsoever, while I'm a nurse who's spent my entire career in health care. And Greg's the one getting all the instructions pertaining to my care. He's actually never missed one of my doctor's appointments, not a single one. When he's on the road, he FaceTimes in. All of a sudden, Greg was forced to become the primary caregiver, not just for me but our whole family. Cancer changed our entire family dynamic for the better, actually, because it forced us to take a team approach where everyone pitched in with the cleaning, cooking, laundry, and everything else. So all of a sudden, Greg and the boys realized how much they hadn't been doing."

Dara Chadwick wrote a great article about this paradigm shift in the family's lives for *CURE* (Cancer Updates, Research, and Education) magazine in May 2019, explaining how Greg got mad and then got busy.

"I went into fight mode," he told Chadwick for that same article quoted at the beginning of this chapter. "We were both very independent people, especially Gina. She's a go-getter, and she wanted to do everything from dishes and laundry to feeding the kids. After her diagnosis, she couldn't."

Greg stresses how much his fellow pilots "pitched in to help, picking up my flights so I could be home with my wife but still get paid. Some were good friends of mine, and some guys I didn't even know," he added. "And Gina's mom and my parents, as well as the parents of other kids, helped get our kids to practices and kept the routine going."

Count Gina Hollenbeck as a firm believer in developing a strong support system as well, one that can support others in addition to herself.

"Everybody's personality is different. But being with people who are experiencing the same thing is a game changer. The key is to bring good stuff to the table, positive stuff whenever possible. 'I had my scan today and I'm clear.' Or 'I have progression,' but plenty of other people in the room have had progression too, and this is what happened and this is what they did. It reminds you that you're not alone in the experience.

"I became president of a group called ALK Positive, named after the specific genetic marker, identified by DNA testing, that I and many lung cancer patients share. We started out as a Facebook page, with me as president, and before you know it, we had fifteen hundred members with active cancer. Representing their interests, we ended up raising over six hundred thousand dollars. But the difference with us was we let the patients, members of our group, decide which research grants to fund with that money. That's true patient empowerment, and it made our members feel they had a direct stake in their own survival."

Gina also got involved with an organization called Courage Through Cancer, through which she met women fighting ovarian, breast, and brain cancers as well as lung. They gathered together for a magazine cover shoot appropriately christened the "Warrior Shoot," since that's what they'd become: warriors in the war against cancer, fighting to save not just their own lives but all those afflicted.

"One of my fellow cover models for the Warrior Shoot was a woman named Terry Trotter, who was suffering from metastatic breast cancer. Terry, it turned out, had started something she called Pink Wig, the point of which was to empower anyone with cancer, starting with breast cancer, since that's what she had. The idea was to take control of your cancer, instead of letting cancer control you, by showing solidarity. In this case that meant giving any woman going through chemo a pink wig. I had a friend at the time being treated for brain cancer, and I asked Terry if I could have a pink wig for her.

"Terry's cancer had returned at the time and she was back on chemo herself. When I came to see her, she was living out of a hospital bed in the living room so she could be close to her daughter. 'I'm so excited you're taking this wig for your friend,' she told me, smiling like all was right with the world. And I can't tell you how much getting that wig meant to my friend. Her whole demeanor changed when I gave it to her. When one of our original Warriors died, we all went to her funeral wearing matching pink wigs. And I also can't tell you how empowering and uplifting it was to be with these women. We had bonded over something all of us wishes we'd never gotten, but that bond was helping us through. Standing at that funeral, I realized not only was I not afraid to die, but I also was not afraid to truly live."

Speaking of truly living, Gina recently sent me a picture of a sweater that was made by one of her ALK Positive family for a new member who was also a new mother. In an enclosed note she said:

"At the time of diagnosis, Brandi was twenty-five and seven months pregnant with her first child. When her doctors figured out that she had lung cancer, they rushed her to start treatment with chemo and an immunotherapy, but because she hoped to maintain her pregnancy, she asked for other options. That was when she was tested to see if her cancer exhibited any biomarkers, just as mine had. When it turned out she was ALK positive too, her treatment was switched to a targeted therapy, since it would give Brandi a better shot at having a positive outcome."

But that only happened because Brandi had asked about other available options, in effect advocating for herself. Brandi delivered her son Colby early and went on to have a second child while taking another targeted drug. Both babies, I'm happy to report, are happy and healthy today.

"Thanks to you, and research conducted by so many," Gina says to me, "in spite of a stage IV lung cancer diagnosis, patients like me and Brandi are not only surviving but thriving. Many women in our group are even having babies while on targeted therapy. It isn't enough for them just to survive; they want to live. And we are going to live in spite of this disease!"

To that same point, at a recent conference Gina was on a panel where the subject of palliative care came up—generally referring to treatment for a serious illness, but often lumped in with end-of-life concerns. Her answer was as demonstrative as her attitude.

"I don't want to talk about palliative care, because I'm not going to die!"

Talk about refusing to quit, talk about being strong, right? But in Gina Hollenbeck's mind, she doesn't see herself as particularly strong.

"I consider myself to be the most blessed and lucky girl alive. Before cancer I didn't see things so clearly as I do now. I feel I've actually figured out how to live."

In many ways, Anita Figueras was typical of the bravery and courage displayed by lung cancer patients. She fought hers for five years until finally succumbing to the disease in June of 2019. Among her many contributions to our community was a wonderful series of posts and interviews highlighting lesser known and discussed aspects of treatment. Here's one specifically dealing with "Building a Support Network When You are a Single Person with Lung Cancer." The interview featured a patient named Karen Loss and appeared on Lungcancer.net in 2017. It is reprinted here with permission.

Karen, please tell us about your connection to lung cancer.

I had no connection to lung cancer at all until, after nearly two years of on again, off again searching for answers to my recurrent "chest attacks" that everyone seemed to think was potentially related to my gall bladder, I was finally sent for a CT scan that showed masses in my right lung and liver. A subsequent needle biopsy in late November of 2012 proved conclusively that I had metastatic lung cancer. I've been battling it ever since then and have chosen to become a patient spokesman and advocate as well.

You are both single and childless, which could pose a big challenge with building a support network when our society is built around nuclear families. Who do you rely on for support?

Literally, from the day I was diagnosed, I made the conscious decision to share my journey with my entire list of friends and family, people with whom I was in email contact. That initially numbered well over 100 people and has grown to about 250 people whom I regularly communicate with regarding my medical circumstances. Some of these people are local and work with me or attend my church, some are family, some are friends in distant places, and now many are also fellow lung cancer patients. I live alone, so I knew it would be up to me to create any support system I might want or need.

You are still working, which is very understandable; you don't have a partner with whom you can share basic living expenses. Are your employer and coworkers part of your support network?

I am very grateful to friends at work who have supported me emotionally during this journey and to management who have given me the leeway necessary to attend myriad medical appointments. They have also been understanding when I need to come in late or otherwise take a break when side effects of some treatments have overcome me. I recognize how lucky I am to be employed by a company that builds flexibility into its work requirements and even allows me to work from home on days when this may be my only reasonable alternative.

As to the single income situation, this is something that can potentially cause a good deal of stress. It's hard enough in this day and age to pay the bills on a single income, but when one adds significant deductibles, drug expenses, and other bills related to cancer treatment, well, it can be daunting. Only recently, I contemplated the possibility of going on disability at least for a time, while I deal with side effects of a difficult treatment regimen, but have determined that it would impact my investment accounts in ways I'm trying to avoid for as long as possible. So, I have opted to tough it out and keep working at figuring out other alternatives to address those nasty side effect issues.

Are you a member of a church? What role does your faith play in your overall support?

Yes, I attend a United Methodist church regularly and feel that my faith ultimately sustains me through this entire experience. It allows me to feel no long-term fear with regard to the fact that my disease is considered a terminal condition because I believe in eternal life…a time when all pain and sickness will be gone and I will live in a new realm of joy with my Lord.

Do you have contingency plans for getting help if you can no longer live independently?

One of my sisters who lives in near proximity to me has agreed to become my caregiver, should that time come when I can no longer care for myself unaided. As a single, independent person, I know this will be difficult for me to deal with, but it is good to know that these plans, however preliminary they may be at this point, are in place.

Have you found ways to use your solitary time that strengthen your emotional well-being? How much do you rely on distractions, such as television?

Well, in all honesty, I watch far too much TV and I web-surf entirely too much also. This is one of the drawbacks of being not only single but an introvert by nature. I really want to get out and be more physically active with such pursuits as hiking, golf, and tennis, but I rarely have anyone to do these things with, so I tend to take the easy way out and relax in front of the TV. I read quite a lot, both fiction and articles, mostly about lung cancer. Oh, and whenever I get the chance, I cheer on the Washington Nationals baseball team. Go Nats!

You are active online, notably with your "Trekking Through Cancerland" Facebook page. What role does advocacy play in your life?

As I have grown more active over the past few years as a patient advocate, I have built a Facebook and Twitter presence. Mostly, in these online settings, I try to share up-to-date happenings in the world of lung cancer research and human-interest stories. My goal is to provide both education and hope to my subscribers. In addition to these outlets, I accept speaking opportunities whenever they present themselves. There are many lung cancer patients around the country, but very few who are available to share firsthand experiences about living and dealing with this disease. I literally feel like this is an obligation, a mission, for me.

What are your thoughts on dating and romance for single people who have stage IV lung cancer?

I believe this is quite individual in nature, but I suspect many single people with stage IV disease probably feel uneasy about starting new romantic relationships. First, the question is always in our minds about how long we may survive, and this leads to wondering if it is fair to put someone in the position of potentially falling in love, with expected heartbreak on the horizon. Second, there is always the uncomfortable question of whether to tell someone right up front about one's disease and risk them fleeing right away, or not telling them for a while until something begins to get serious and risk them feeling a lack of trust as a result.

One friend has told me she plans to be bold and blunt. If they run away, good for 'em. She'll move on to the next until the right connection is made. That's a good outlook, but sometimes harder to put into practice than it sounds.

Is there anything you feel you miss out on as you go through your lung cancer experience because you are single and unattached?

Fortunately, as an introvert, I am generally comfortable spending most of my time alone. That said, however, I do miss having someone at hand to talk to, not only about lung cancer but just about the mundane things in life. Sometimes that is even more important in order to divert one's mind away from the challenges and trials relating to ongoing treatments and side effects.

I miss having a companion to travel with. When I was diagnosed four and a half years ago and learned of the bleak statistics surrounding lung cancer, particularly stage IV disease, I thought a good bit about taking life by the horns and checking off bucket list items. After all, more than most, people in my shoes know that time is of the essence. But, it's so much more fun to experience things with others rather than solo, and as a single person, it can be a challenge to find partners for big adventures.

Do you have any final thoughts about being single while battling lung cancer?

I would encourage others in similar circumstances to be proactive. If you need to find transportation to and from appointments, don't wait for others to offer. Seek help. Find a Stephen Ministry in your community. They'll help at no cost to you. If you find yourself too sick to make your meals or care for your house and yard, talk to your minister. Ask your friends for help. If you just need someone to talk to, pick up the phone or sit down at your computer and make the contacts.

In my experience, very few people approach me. I tell myself it is because they see me as highly independent and it simply doesn't occur to them. Whatever the reason, I know that as a single person, it's not likely to happen if I don't make it happen. Don't be timid. Don't be afraid. As Nike says, "Just do it!"

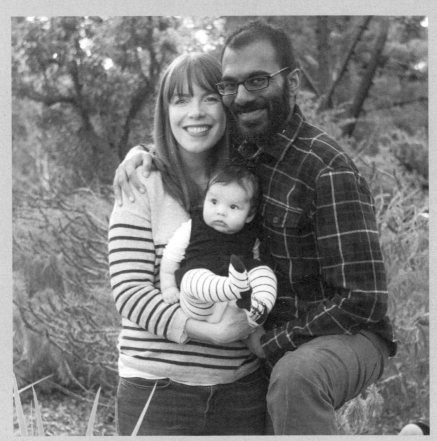

Photo by Suszi McFadden

2

Lucy and Paul Kalanithi

I *flipped through the CT scan images, the diagnosis obvious: the lungs were matted with innumerable tumors, the spine deformed, a full lobe of the liver obliterated. Cancer, widely disseminated. I was a neurosurgical resident entering my final year of training. Over the last six years, I'd examined scores of such scans, on the off chance that some procedure might benefit the patient. But this scan was different: it was my own.*

So opens *When Breath Becomes Air*, Dr. Paul Kalanithi's heart-wrenching chronicle of his own life and ultimate death to lung cancer, that tugged on my heart strings and then tied them into knots. He and his wife, Lucy, had brought a beautiful little girl, Cady, into the world eight months before his passing. Though Cady has no actual memory of her father, Lucy is determined not to let her forget him. When I stop by for a visit, I notice the photographs of Paul that adorn their Northern California home. But it was something else that impressed me even more: an entire picture book of Paul that sits right alongside similar tomes that feature the likes of Elmo and Peppa Pig.

"Cady talks about Paul a lot," Lucy says about her daughter, who's now four years old. "He's like a character she's learning about through pictures and stories I tell her. Recently, she had to do a family portrait in preschool, and she drew one picturing 'mom, dad, and baby me.' She knows everyone has a dad and it's not like she doesn't have one. But she drew herself as 'baby me,' because she was a baby when Paul was still alive. 'I was a baby with my daddy,' she says. The fact that he's her father doesn't stop being true because he's gone."

Lucy penned the epilogue for *When Breath Becomes Air*, which Paul managed to finish but wasn't published until nine months after his death. And it's become for her kind of what the picture book of Paul is for Cady, in that it helps her remember the man she loved so much instead of merely not forgetting him.

"Paul says in the book a lot of people who get sick ask, Why me?" she says, echoing the same point made by Gina Hollenbeck. "Well, the answer is, Why not me? Paul was a doctor, a brain surgeon who saw terrible things happening to people all the time. He had a firm grasp on the concept of what it means to be human, of making sense of the world through our fragile, finite bodies. Death is a fact of life, yet it's so hard to grasp. So you find meaning in your life, both despite and because you're mortal. More than anything, the book made me less afraid, and I want it to do the same for so many others out there who are just like me."

Lucy doesn't look scared at all. Her eyes are blue and wide, in contrast to Cady's, which are big and brown, just like her father's.

"When I brush her teeth in the morning, I think about Paul. She and I look different because of him, because he's still inside her. I think about that a lot. People ask me if I ever had second thoughts about bringing a child into the world in Paul's final months. I tell them I can't imagine not having done it. Even then, he was more sure about being a parent than I was, despite the fact that our big worry was that having a child would make dying more painful, because he'd have to say good-bye to her too, not just me."

One chapter of my life seemed to have ended; perhaps the whole book was closing. Instead of being the pastoral figure aiding a life transition, I found myself the sheep, lost and confused. Severe illness wasn't life-altering, it was life-shattering. It felt less like an epiphany—a piercing burst of light, illuminating What Really Matters—and more like someone had just firebombed the path forward…. My life had been building potential, potential that would now go unrealized. I had planned to do so much, and I had come so close. I was physically debilitated, my imagined future and my personal identity collapsed, and I faced the same existential quandaries my patients faced. The lung cancer diagnosis was confirmed. My carefully planned and hard-won future no longer existed. Death, so familiar to me in my work, was now paying a personal visit. Here we were, finally face-to-face, and yet nothing about it seemed recognizable. Standing at the crossroads where I should have been able to see and follow the footprints of the countless patients I had treated over the years. I saw instead only a blank, a harsh, vacant, gleaming white desert, as if a sandstorm had erased all trace of familiarity.

That's the man whom Lucy loved until the day he died. A doctor with magnificent dreams dashed, who went from asking *Why me?* to *Why not me?* and managed to squeeze a lifetime into his final days as a result.

"*When Breath Becomes Air,*" she writes in the epilogue, "is in a sense, unfinished, derailed by Paul's rapid decline, but that is an essential component of its truth, of the reality Paul faced. During the last year of his life, Paul wrote relentlessly, fueled by purpose, motivated by a ticking clock. He started with midnight bursts when he was still a neurosurgery chief resident, softly tapping away on his laptop as he lay next to me in bed; later he spent afternoons in his recliner, drafted paragraphs in his oncologist's waiting room, took phone calls from his editor while chemotherapy dripped into his veins, carried his silver laptop everywhere he went. When his fingertips developed painful fissures because of his chemotherapy, we found seamless, silver-lined gloves that allowed use of a trackpad and keyboard. Strategies for retaining the mental focus needed to write, despite the punishing fatigue of progressive cancer, was the primary subject of his palliative-care appointments. He was determined to keep writing."

Just like Lucy is determined to keep living. I look at her across the table and wished I had more answers for her. I'd first met both Paul and her just after Lucy learned she was pregnant. The joy of that was tempered considerably by the fact Paul knew he was dying, but I'm not sure I've ever met anyone fuller of life, as if he were channeling the essence of his unborn child, secure in the notion he could leave this world knowing that he'd left his mark in the form of a legacy beyond books and patients.

Gazing at Lucy, I realized I didn't have any answers for her because she hadn't posed any questions. And, in point of fact, I think our relationship was as much about her helping me, if not even more. I had gotten sick, and now I was better. She had lost her husband and he wasn't coming back. Her inner strength, mental and spiritual, is a force to behold. The way she keeps memories of Paul alive for her daughter is the best therapy in the world for her as well as Cady.

A clinical assistant professor of medicine at the Stanford University School of Medicine, Lucy met Paul at Yale Medical School in 2003 and they married three years later. They'd been together for a decade when Paul was diagnosed; that left them with only a few cherished years together. Even though they knew they were up against a ticking clock, they made the decision to have a child, and the couple made every one of those months, weeks, and days count in their time together with their newborn.

"Paul's memoir," Lucy tells me, "ends with a particularly poignant message to Cady that's now framed in her bedroom at home: 'When you come to one of the many moments in life where you must give an account of yourself, provide a ledger of what you have been and done and meant to the world, do not, I pray, discount that you filled a dying man's days with a sated joy, a joy unknown to me in all my prior years, a joy that does not hunger for more and more but rests, satisfied. In this time, right now, that is an enormous thing.'"

The huge success of the book serves as great comfort to Lucy. But its lessons are hard ones, and time has done little to soften the life-changing sense that a lung cancer diagnosis brings. Thousands of people seated across from their doctor get that same news every single day, and understanding the strength of people like Lucy and Paul Kalanithi offers the best recipe for hope there is.

"The success of Paul's book is kind of bittersweet, because he wasn't here to see it. I wish I could tell him about it, wish I could tell him about Cady. That's the hardest thing about being diagnosed with any serious illness: you realize you may never see the fruits of your labors. You live your life pursuing the things that are so important to you and when you're first diagnosed, you suddenly realize your entire identity vested in your future self, who you imagine you will be, has evaporated. You're the very same person you were five minutes before in one respect, but also an entirely different one in another. How long have I got left? Who am I still and what can I still have? How should I spend my time, living with so much uncertainty?

"Paul went back to work because that was so important to his identity, who he was as a person. That created this void when he wasn't able to physically handle being a doctor anymore. So he turned his attention to having Cady and to writing. And the writing felt so good, became his purpose, lent meaning to what he was doing. Victor Frankel once said something like, 'He who has a why to live can bear almost any how.' Paul's struggle was with keeping his life meaningful, which was where the writing came in."

Lucy looks at me with eyes that can best be described as soulful. That's not a physical trait so much as the experience she imparts in every gaze, almost like in looking ahead she's also looking back at the same time. The past and the present wondrously unified in another inclination that defines her strength. She hasn't moved on, no; she's simply moved forward.

"The book became Paul's purpose, and I was so happy I was able to continue that by going on tour and meeting so many people who'd been touched by his words. That was so helpful to me because it gave me a reason to talk about Paul, and that's when I still felt his presence in my life. When somebody dies, you don't stop thinking about them. You still love them. I remember this story Sheryl Sandberg told after losing her husband about going to a dinner party with several couples who were longtime friends. They went around the table swapping stories of how they'd met their spouses, but then skipped right over her, as if her husband's death had erased his very existence."

What is it, though, that Lucy wants *When Breath Becomes Air* to achieve? I ask her. What is it about the book, besides the memories of Paul it rekindles, that makes it as important to her today as the day it was published?

"That's really hard to put into words. But the book is bigger than me, bigger even than Paul. I want patients and families to read it. The lessons people learn from your cancer are different from what you learned from your cancer. How do you go forward as a different version of yourself? Who am I now? How do I accept this? How do I go forward with this life, thinking about myself in an entirely different manner that I did before? Amputees often talk of still feeling their lost appendage, like a phantom limb. For cancer patients, that's more like a phantom future. Your new reality changes the way you interact with life, with the world, and I want Paul's book to help other patients adjust to that new reality."

Before my cancer was diagnosed, I knew that someday I would die, but I didn't know when. After the diagnosis, I knew that someday I would die, but I didn't know when. But now I knew it acutely. The problem wasn't really a scientific one. The fact of death is unsettling. Yet there is no other way to live.

While Paul looms large in Lucy's life, he'd told her on multiple occasions prior to his death that he wanted her to remarry. Since he died, she has formed a close relationship with a man named John who'd lost his wife and was raising two young boys. I asked her how she knew it was time, that she was ready.

"Let me think about that for a second. It was two years after Paul died, and John and I just started writing to each other after we met briefly while I was on tour for Paul's book. It wasn't like I went on Match.com or something. And I had to check in with myself once it started happening, once it was clear we were attracted to each other. People talk about the timeline for grief. You get advice like don't do anything, make no big decisions, for a year. But it's not that predictable. There's no book to read or boilerplate to follow. You just have to trust yourself, that it's natural to take two steps forward and one step back. Whatever you're feeling is okay. Because John's wife had also died, it was really easy to talk about the experience we shared. We intuitively understood the fact that you can love two people at the same time. He was never going to stop loving his wife, and I was never going to stop loving Paul."

Lucy broke up with John after a year or so. It was a long-distance relationship, and their time together was just what each of them needed when they'd first met. Since then, she bought a new house. After Paul's death, she couldn't imagine moving out of the home she'd shared with him, but she decided to relocate to a neighborhood near the school Cady would be attending a few years down the road. It wasn't so much closing one door, literally and figuratively, as opening a new one.

Doctors, Paul wrote in *When Breath Becomes Air*, need hope too. And more than anything in his final days, Paul found that hope in the daughter he knew he wouldn't live to see grow up.

"Cady loves all things that her dad loved," Lucy tells me.

You'd think maybe she'd say that tearfully, but instead the words emerge ahead of a reflective smile born of a deep appreciation of the past and a view forward into the future.

"I tell her little things about Paul. One day she wanted to wear mismatched shoes to preschool. I told her, 'Your dad used to do that. Put them on.' So she looked at me and said, 'This is what me and my dad do.'"

I ask Lucy what advice she has to other survivors after a loved one has succumbed to cancer or any disease.

"I tell them what you once told me," she answers, a glint flashing in her eyes. "That it can be lonely facing the new normal, even when you're not alone. That it's good to have a protective buffer when you can be strong for the people you need to be strong for and then go and secretly cry. Bonnie, you also told me about simply sitting around a table with friends and articulating the thing that scares you the most. Then you have a place to start. Sometimes, there's nothing anyone can say that can make things better. The pain is so acute at the beginning, so all-consuming that it seems it will never go away. But it does, it does get better. And loving the person who's gone never goes away, nor should it."

I want to hug her in that moment. Looking across the table with the sun streaming in through the windows and brightening her youthful features, I realize Lucy Kalanithi has just articulated something straight out of the Living Room.

"I expected to feel only empty and heartbroken after Paul died," she wrote in that beautiful epilogue from *When Breath Becomes Air*. "It never occurred to me that you could love someone the same way after he was gone, that I would continue to feel such love and gratitude alongside the terrible sorrow, the grief so heavy that at times I shiver and moan under the weight of it. Paul is gone, and I miss him acutely nearly every moment, but I somehow feel I'm still taking part in the life we created together. 'Bereavement is not the truncation of married love,' C. S. Lewis wrote, 'but one of its regular phases—like the honeymoon. What we want is to live our marriage well and faithfully through that phase too.' Caring for our daughter, nurturing relationships with family, publishing this book, pursuing meaningful work, visiting Paul's grave, grieving and honoring him, persisting…my love goes on—lives on—in a way I'd never expected."

Dr. Pasi Jänne is the kind of physician you want to see when you're looking for lung cancer treatment options, when you're looking for hope. Working out of Boston's Dana-Farber Cancer Institute, Dr. Jänne is on the cutting edge of therapies aimed at extending life and turning lung cancer into a manageable disease. Here's Part One of his thoughts on the state of lung cancer treatment today.

When I started out, and for a number of years afterward, there was a stigma associated with lung cancer, a stigma we work very hard to dispel. When you read in the obituaries that someone died of cancer, and the particular type isn't mentioned, it's usually lung cancer because of the misplaced shame associated with the disease, and that's a barrier to getting people the help and care they need. In large part that same stigma, the myth that lung cancer is strictly a smoker's cancer, was behind the lack of funding for the disease. The good news is that's not the case anymore. It's changing, but we have to continue to be patient.

I rotate between patient care and clinically based research. The patient part keeps it real for me, keeps my fingers on the pulse and puts a human face on the problems my research is trying to solve. When you move away from that approach, when you don't see patients, you lose what it's like to be fighting this battle day to day in the trenches. Treating patients is an inspiration and reality check for me at the same time, a reminder that despite all the clinical subsets and therapies that are out there, people are still dying. That's a constant reminder to me that makes me work harder and think harder about how we can do better.

The other issue is that any treatment model you generate is only as good as the clinical scenario it came from. Being directly involved with patients allows me to see firsthand the side effects of the therapies we develop for lung cancer and the relative resistance to the drug on behalf of the patients suffering from the disease. This combination of disciplines isn't even possible outside the United States, where it's basically an either-or situation. I'm able to take findings directly from the lab to the clinic, because I've seen what's possible in the clinic and enjoy an appreciation for what's possible in a human as opposed to a mouse.

Twenty years ago, the practice of oncology was easier, easier in the sense that oncologists tended to be jacks-of-all-trades who treated a bunch of cancers, even all of them. Everything's different now, because the huge increase in the number of therapies for cancers across the board and the nuances associated with them make it impossible for any doctor to stay ahead of the curve. We've entered the era of specialization where the information curve is not only steep, it's constantly changing. And things are changing so fast in terms of testing and treatment that when I go to conferences, I can't imagine going to all the sessions or even most of them. I only go to the lung cancer sessions.

The other thing, another positive, is that an oncologist in rural Nebraska is no longer limited by a lack of specialization and pure distance from top cancer centers like Dana-Farber. They can now convene digital tumor boards (a group of doctors and other health care providers with different specialties that meets to determine the best possible cancer treatment and care plan for an individual patient) to discuss the patient's treatment and prognosis. They can request e-consults. I had a patient from Syracuse come to me and I recommended something, a treatment protocol, they could take back to their oncologist there who wasn't a lung cancer specialist.

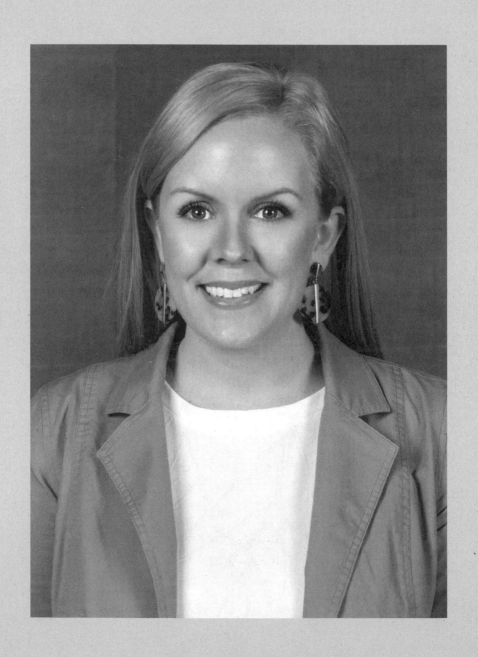

3

Taylor Bell Duck

*I*t doesn't make sense. How can a former Division I athlete who never *smoked get lung cancer?*

Your Cancer Game Plan, a wonderfully proactive website dedicated to helping those battling cancer, has a program they call With Love, Me in which survivors pen letters to themselves chronicling their disease. The passage above opens thirty-one-year-old Taylor Duck's especially inspiring, and informative, letter that's typical of the kind of support we created the Living Room to provide.

You just started dating a guy! Talk about not great timing. Your life just changed significantly and even though you don't look physically sick, you are. Make sure your friends and family understand the severity of your diagnosis and set boundaries around what you will and will not talk about. When you're scared, show it. When you feel badly, say it. Don't lose hope.

Just like Taylor never did. Every time we talk, soccer enters the conversation.

"Playing soccer was the best feeling in the world," she told me recently when we met at a restaurant near the hospital she works out of in North Carolina as an administrator for Vidant Health. "Being on the field made me feel I was super alive."

Taylor is as beautiful today as the day she first reached out to me, looking for a way to help others in the wake of her own successful treatment. Her blonde hair tumbles just past her shoulders, and her easy smile flashes often. She still looks like an athlete, even the slightest motion graceful, her long, loping stride making it easy to picture her racing up the soccer field and nailing goals in the top corner of the net. She'd been playing since she was four years old, a true competitor even back then who attacked the ball with relentless passion. She played on elite youth teams throughout her school years, ultimately realizing her dream to play for a Division I college at East Carolina. Every living second, Taylor is fond of saying, was dedicated to the sport.

She showed up for preseason camp her freshman year in great shape, ready to compete for a starting spot. Only she couldn't pass a challenging but relatively routine fitness test. No matter how many times she tried, she couldn't finish this endurance test, only able to get through about half of it. Then she started experiencing numbness and loss of feeling in her toes, to go with a worsening shortness of breath.

"I thought I couldn't have lung cancer because I never smoked or even been around secondhand smoke. And I was only eighteen years old."

The first doctors she saw felt the same way, believing she was suffering from recurring pneumonia or bronchitis. That's what they treated her for, and she seemed to be getting better. Then her symptoms returned, having worsened. This time a larger battery of tests was ordered, and the doctor shocked her with the results.

"You've got a small spot on your lung that's concerning."

But a nurse begged to differ. "It's not a spot, it's a mass," she told Taylor after the doctor had left the room.

"I was in a state of shock," Taylor says, recalling that day as if it were yesterday. "The truth is I hadn't been feeling all that well for a really long time. I kept brushing off the symptoms because I was so healthy and a collegiate-level athlete too. How could something so serious be wrong with me? I got up and went to the gym in high school every morning with my dad at five a.m. I did everything right and I kept telling myself it would pass. But, of course, it didn't."

Develop a thick skin and come up with clever things to say when people ask "did you smoke?" her With Love, Me letter continues. *"Remind your friends and family that even though the situation is harsh, it doesn't have to consume you or them."*

How can it not, though? That's the one thing all cancer patients share. The battle to beat the disease becomes all-consuming because it has to. I remember reading stories from British survivors of World War II telling of what it was like enduring the constant barrage of German bombing. That didn't just dominate their lives, it became their lives. It's the same thing when you're fighting cancer, bombs going off in a body that seems to have turned against you.

Taylor reached out to me through the foundation I'd started with my husband, Tony, after she'd weathered the storm and climbed out of the figurative shelter she'd taken refuge in through the duration of her fight.

"Remember," she reflects today about our initial contact, "how I'd already gotten involved with the Lung Cancer Initiative of North Carolina, but I felt my story was so powerful I needed to share it beyond the state? We started chatting, emailing, and talking about the changing face of cancer, how more and more young women were getting diagnosed and how none of them had ever smoked. I wanted to speak up and use my voice. I couldn't speak through my play on the soccer field anymore, so I found a new voice."

Taylor calls the decision to give up soccer, mandated by her inability to compete physically anymore, the hardest thing she'd ever done. It had defined her life for fourteen years. Now cancer was providing that definition instead.

"But in a good way after I beat it," she elaborates. "I made it a personal mission to defy the stigmas and stereotypes, like only smokers get this disease."

The advocacy, which began in her undergraduate years at East Carolina University, morphed into the career path she ultimately chose. As of this writing, Taylor serves as physician outreach manager of market development for Vidant Health, based in Greenville, North Carolina, a position from which she's able to positively affect the lives and outcomes for those, like her, who've been struck by illness.

"Vidant Health is one of the largest hospital systems in the country, consisting of eight community hospitals. My job is to call on physicians across the state who aren't part of our system to educate them on our system of care. I introduce them to our physicians and do a deep dive into their referral patterns toward bringing them into our family of doctors, at least in terms of referring patients to specialists, particularly in oncology. I want to give doctors outside our system an opportunity to provide the absolute best health care for their patients.

"I've always had an interest in health care," Taylor continues, flashing the smile that is no less broad since her days on the soccer field. "But I was a political science and history major. I was going to go to Washington and change the world, which seemed even more apt in the wake of my surviving lung cancer. And I did go to Washington as part of something called the National Coalition for Cancer Survivorship, but I just didn't like the lifestyle or the bureaucracy. And more to the point, I didn't get the sense I'd be able to accomplish anything meaningful working that track. But I wasn't looking for something clinical. I wanted to make an appreciable difference in patient outcomes by improving the care they received."

I ask Taylor what she means by that.

"Well, being a patient myself has really helped my outreach and engagement. I bring a unique perspective to the table, but I don't want to be the girl who's always talking about her own diagnosis. I have the opportunity to change and make a difference in patient care, away from the clinical side and the bedside. I take the lessons I learned as a patient and apply them to my work as an administrator."

Like what?

"The first key, the first priority, is quick access to care. How long is the lag between diagnosis and time to treatment? I was treated at Duke University Medical Center, which just might be the finest facility anywhere when it comes to thoracic surgery and oncology. So I know what the best standard of care looks like, and as an administrator, my goal is to do everything I can to make sure every patient has access to that. I have a friend whose mom, due to fragmented care, had trouble getting a diagnosis and then waited six weeks to start treatment at a point waiting even six days might have been too long. And the national average between diagnosis and treatment is forty-seven days, basically seven weeks. In Vidant Health's system, the average lag is five days. That's the standard of care I'm trying to bring to every part of North Carolina. I want all lung cancer patients, all cancer patients in general, to get the best and most up-to-date treatment, not something ten years old dispensed by a practitioner unaware of the latest targeted therapies, immunotherapies, and clinical trials. Everyone who's sick deserves the absolute best care they can get."

"So," I ask her, "what are Taylor Duck's rules for just-diagnosed patients?"

She answers without pause for thought, as if she's already done all the thinking she needs to do on the subject based on personal experience. "First, never go to an appointment alone. You need an extra set of ears, because the deluge of information you're being given is overwhelming and it's impossible to take it all in. I personally kept a tote bag filled with every bill, every notice, every document I ever received about my cancer so I'd know where to look if I ever needed to find something. Second, get a second opinion. That's really important, especially when eighty-five percent of cancer patients are being treated at a community oncology setting in which the oncologist may be treating all cancers instead of specializing in one.

"Speaking of overwhelming, the data on lung cancer alone is so great it's hard to keep up with it all even if you are a specialist, never mind if you're not. Things end up falling through the cracks, and patients can tumble down after them. Oh, and get a copy of your test results and scans in case you need to share them. Electronic medical records don't always communicate from system to system all that well. So you want to have your records available in case there's an emergency or you just want another opinion.

"I also think it's important to advocate for yourself, because you know your body better than anyone else. And so if you feel like something isn't right, push until you have answers. There's no reason somebody shouldn't feel their toes or train as hard as I did and not be successful. I think what's also important is to use your support team around you, and when they're trying to advocate for you, to listen to them as well. There were several times where my mom spoke with my provider and said, 'Please order an additional test. We have a strong family history.' And they brushed her off, and I kind of was like, 'Oh, I've got the crazy mom trying to tell the doctor how to practice medicine.' But I think that when you have a team that's able to support you, you should let them.

"I also stress doing research in terms of an advocacy standpoint, which means reaching out to folks like you, Bonnie, and making use of the resources available from your foundation. And come to the Living Room," she adds, flashing another smile. "But you also need a support system to navigate your system of care. I saw this firsthand after my own diagnosis. It turned out the best thoracic surgeon in the world was right here at Duke, Dr. Thomas D'Amico. But his office said he was leaving in the morning to teach in China and it would be three or four weeks until they could get me in. So my mom got in touch with someone in our church who'd had lung cancer and was being treated by Dr. D'Amico."

"Let me text him real quick," the woman said, pulling out her phone.

A YOUNG GIRL FROM OUR CHURCH HAS LUNG CANCER AND NEEDS TO SEE YOU.

The response from Dr. D'Amico came back in seconds.

WHERE IS SHE? CAN SHE COME IN TONIGHT?

"And I did. We drove to Duke immediately, and Dr. D'Amico saw us that evening. He became my oncologist, overseeing all of my care. He's a physician who looks at a patient as a whole, what I used to be able to do and what I wanted to do now. And he also saw in me someone who could contribute to a higher cause. Maybe three or four months later, when I saw him again, I was wreck. I was sitting in his office instead of on spring break with my friends."

"'I know you're upset, Taylor,'" Dr. D'Amico said to me. "'What's happened to you isn't fair. But the blessing here is that you can share your story with others. You're beautiful, smart, and articulate, and I need you to do this for me, to go out and share your story.'

"This was the godfather of thoracic surgery asking me to do something for him. I mean, he was like God to me, and he's been a mentor ever since. And that's what this community's all about—paying it forward and back."

Look for the "gifts" from your new diagnosis—maybe it's that you get to slow down, or that you now appreciate the small things that you used to overlook, Taylor's With Love, Me letter goes on. *Or maybe you meet the nicest guy in the world who will stand by your side, coach you through your recovery and one day he will become your husband. Don't doubt God's timing.*

"And that's what pretty much what happened with you, isn't it?" I ask her.

She smiles, saying nothing because she doesn't have to.

There's a video featuring Taylor on the Your Cancer Game Plan site, appropriately called "Switching Plays." It opens with the Taylor of today dribbling a soccer ball in a moment that rekindles old glories.

"It's the greatest feeling in the world" is the first thing you hear her say in voiceover. "Being on the field made me feel like I was super alive. When you spend your life dedicated to a game and then one day you say, 'You know what? I'm not going to do this anymore,' that's a really hard decision to make. But something wasn't right with me. If I did all this right, then what went wrong?"

In addition to chronicling Taylor's love of the game and rise to stardom, the video introduces us to her then boyfriend, Robert, a high school football coach at the time. They'd been dating for only two weeks prior to her diagnosis.

"Robert really was my coach throughout the entire process," Taylor continues in her narration of the video, both of us getting teary-eyed as we watch it for the umpteenth time, but this time together, "in terms of helping me walk through the steps of initial diagnosis and then helping me throughout surgery and recovery. Making sure I was getting up and walking and doing the things I was supposed to be doing."

I get teary-eyed again, thinking of how much I can relate to that, thanks to my husband, Tony. How he was there for and with me every step of the way through my own diagnosis and treatment, and how important it is to have a Tony or a Robert in your life when you're dealing with lung cancer, or any cancer for that matter.

We go back to watching the video.

"Taylor really found her voice on the soccer field," her sister says near the end. "That was where she put up a dominant face. And for a while after her diagnosis, it was like, What's she going to do now that she isn't playing anymore? But I think that since she was diagnosed she's found another voice."

"You've grown a lot," she continues after turning toward Taylor, who's seated next to her on the living room couch for the filming of the video. "You had to."

"I've made it a personal mission of mine to speak up and educate people about the disease," Taylor picks up from there. "To really try to defy the stigma that only smokers get this disease, because it can happen to anyone. I believe it's important that anytime I get the opportunity to speak up and talk about it that I should. I'm not upset about the way my college experience went. I'm actually really grateful for it because it taught me what's important in life: it's relationships, your family, and your friends."

Taylor and her mother, Nancy, recorded a video for CURE Connections, a wonderful video site that helps answer patients' questions about their cancer diagnosis. The second serialized segment addresses another common trait: the guilt experienced by cancer patients and caregivers alike.

"Before Taylor was diagnosed, the surgeon said to her, 'I bet you haven't been well for a while,'" Nancy says. "My husband is able to laugh about that now. He's let go of the guilt, but he did have some guilt initially because there was some time that Taylor would stand on the soccer field with her hands on her hips. And we were filming her because she was going to play college soccer, and my husband would tease her and say, 'You know you can't stand on the soccer field with your hands on the hips.' Well, in hindsight the reason she was doing that was because she couldn't breathe and she was trying to get air in her lungs. And so we now joke about that. But for a while, once we realized this was a lung cancer diagnosis, there was a lot of guilt. But we allowed ourselves to forgive ourselves."

Taylor's thirty-one now and is ten years cancer-free. She's married to Robert and a while back celebrated receiving a master's degree in public administration. And as a health care professional, she has a different perspective on what it's going to take to continue making dramatic inroads in treatments of all cancers, but especially lung cancer, the greatest killer of them all. I reach across the table and squeeze her hand and find myself not wanting to let go. Given the fragility of life, if I let go, she might slip away and be gone. Taylor returns my grasp, a look in her eye telling me she's feeling the very same thing. So there we are, two survivors of lung cancer who defied the odds, afraid to let go of each other because we're stronger together.

"There has to be a group of individuals involved for us to beat this disease," Taylor says. "Patients, health care providers, advocacy organizations. Without everyone having a seat at the table, we won't be able to do this, and that table includes the pharmaceutical industry."

That Your Cancer Game Plan website referenced earlier was actually created by the pharmaceutical company Merck to give lung patients a portal to make a game plan for their treatment and diagnosis and to help navigate that journey. That included the With Love, Me program in which Taylor participated. For all the negative publicity big pharmaceutical companies like Merck attract, they genuinely do great, at times even miraculous, work. And so many people owe their lives to the drugs now available that weren't just a few years back.

"Merck is providing great resources for patients to be more involved in their treatment," Taylor says. "To put a human face on the disease, they've brought me in to speak to seven hundred people at their headquarters in New Jersey. They wouldn't do that if they weren't genuinely interested in patient outcomes, and not just in making the most money possible off their drugs."

You might say Taylor's experience with lung cancer and the health care industry has been all about breaking down stigma and mythologies, from being diagnosed at the age of eighteen to talking straight about Big Pharma's role in bringing new drugs to the marketplace that can further extend lives and make lung cancer a manageable disease.

It's okay to have a life! Taylor's With Love, Me letter concludes. *Enjoy the things that bring you joy. Everyone processes a diagnosis differently, and there is no right or wrong way to do this. Want to pull the "cancer card"? Pull it anytime you want.*

Author's note: Taylor is now working for Merck Pharmaceuticals.

FIFTH GRADER RUNS 50 5K'S IN 50 DAYS
FOR GRANDPA'S LUNG CANCER

That was the headline that greeted me a foggy day in October of 2018 on the website of KPIX 5, the Bay Area's local CBS affiliate.

The article it referenced told the story of Niall McDermott, a local ten-year-old boy who wanted to do something special for his grandfather who was battling lung cancer at the time. Niall had been particularly inspired by an athlete who completed fifty triathlons over fifty consecutive days. Niall's goal:

"I wanted to do fifty 5Ks in fifty days," he told KPIX.

The boy's quest started with a 5K race in nearby Golden Gate Park. That was followed by running another 5K the following day, and again the day after. But even after a week straight, Niall's father, Ryan, still harbored doubts about whether his son could keep it up.

"No, I thought it was very unlikely," he told KPIX. "Ten-year-olds are fantastic, but they embark on a lot of things that they don't finish."

Not Niall. He kept at it, never taking a day off no matter how he felt or how bad the weather was. Since his grandfather wasn't about to quit his fight against lung cancer, the boy wasn't about to abandon his goal, even as he kept raising money at every turn to donate to support his grandfather's cause.

"He never complained a single day, said he didn't want to do it, or he's too tired or something hurt," his mother, Maggie, told KPIX. "He was just ready to go every day. I'm amazed. I've never really known a kid to do something like this, personally. I'm proud to be his mom."

Then came day number fifty, the final one in his quest, in which he was joined by a friend in a local swim-and-run competition to complete his final 5K.

"I was thinking, 'I'm gonna finish this and I can do it, and when I finish it, I won't have to do it anymore,'" he told KPIX just after crossing the finish line.

The $4,000 that Niall raised, a princely sum in honor of his grandfather, was donated to the Bonnie J. Addario Lung Cancer Foundation, prior to our merger with the Lung Cancer Alliance to become the GO2 Foundation for Lung Cancer, toward crossing another finish line: making lung cancer a manageable, infinitely more survivable disease.

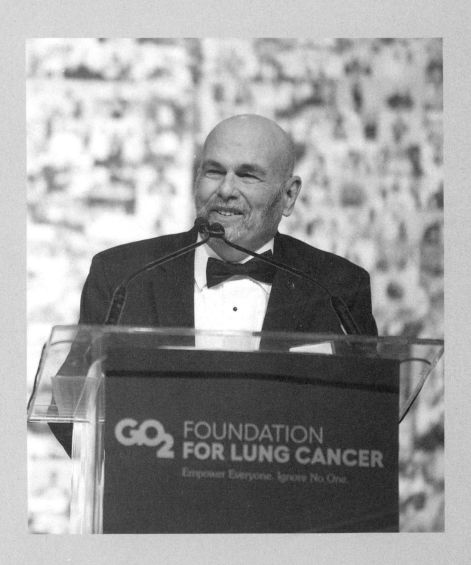

4

Don Stranathan

Ironically enough, Don Stranathan is only alive today because he had to go to prison in 2009.

Yes, you read that right, but not for the reasons you're probably thinking.

"One of the mandatory requirements of volunteering at San Quentin is a medical clearance exam to ensure you are healthy enough to work with the inmates," he told the *ASCO* (American Society of Clinical Oncology) *Post* in May 2017. "To my astonishment, I wasn't as healthy as I thought. In fact, the results from imaging scans, blood tests, and a tissue biopsy showed I had stage IV non-small cell adenocarcinoma. I was given eight to twelve months to live."

We're both in Washington for meetings and decide to meet for dinner at the Capital Grille on Pennsylvania Avenue, across the street from the Federal Trade Commission and across the corner from the Newseum. It's his favorite restaurant in the city, and I know I won't be able to get even within grasping distance of the bill because that's the way Don is.

"I had gotten a routine chest X-ray in 2006 to make sure I didn't have tuberculosis that showed a suspicious lesion on my left lung. The doctors said let's just watch it and right up until my diagnosis three years later, I had no symptoms. A week before my biopsy I hiked to the top of Mount Tam. After twenty-one miles, I was a little short of breath but attributed it to age, given that I was in my mid-fifties. A follow-up chest X-ray had shown the lesion had grown, and a week later a biopsy revealed my bronchus tube was ninety percent blocked. That had actually kept my lung from collapsing. I had a follow-up PET scan in June of 2009 which showed warm [often an indicator of tumor activity] and revealed that another tumor had showed up. The tumor was difficult to reach for a biopsy and after some literal hits and misses, they managed to snip off enough to tell me there was a ninety-five percent chance it was cancer.

"I was floored. I had totally changed my lifestyle twenty years before, quit drinking and smoking when I was thirty-four. But at forty-eight years old they found I had an enlarged heart and told me I was two years away from a heart transplant. That was all I needed to hear to change my diet entirely, then got into hiking and an exercise program. Two years later, when I was supposed to be ready for that heart transplant, I was climbing mountains. I had beaten the heart condition, so I figured I could beat lung cancer too."

The server comes and pours bottled water for both of us, mine sparkling and Don's flat. He asks us if we need more time with the menus and we tell him we do. Around us, the tables are filling up, and it seems like every time someone enters the dining room, heads turn to spot which recognizable political figure it might be. Nobody bothers looking our way, which suits me just fine.

"So ten years after being diagnosed, you're still alive," I say to Don. "Tell me what you believe is responsible for that."

"My feeling from the beginning was that I needed to be my own advocate. Not long after my diagnosis, I met a guy in spin class named John who had the same lung cancer I did and had been diagnosed two years earlier. He asked what treatment they were looking at for me and I gave him the rundown. 'Why aren't you getting the latest?' he asked, referring to a drug that attacks tumors by shutting off their blood supply. I went back to the doctors, pushed for that drug, and got it. I believed strongly that I had to be my own strongest advocate, but I know other patients are comfortable letting caregivers handle more of that chore. In my case, there was no one in my life at the time I wanted to burden with that, and I preferred advocating for myself anyway. I think that's critical."

Because he's now a ten-year lung cancer survivor, the trim and fit-looking Don says people reach out to him from all over the world. That isn't unusual in itself because, thankfully, they reach out to me too. It's the most important thing a just-diagnosed lung cancer patient can do because, as Don says, you don't know what you don't know, and that means finding someone who does. Someone who can offer knowledge and comfort. That might seem like small consolation, but all consolation is important when you've just been told you have lung cancer.

"I'm not a doctor," Don says, "so I'm not going to give anyone medical advice. But I know the questions you should ask your oncologist, like, 'What kind of mutations do I have? Are there any targeted or new immunotherapies I'm eligible for?' Beyond that, for me the best way to get through your hardest times is to help others get through theirs. I'm involved twenty-four/seven in supporting other people. Those connections help me stay in touch with and meet some of the top doctors in the country specializing in lung cancer. But what I stress more than anything is what I just told you: be your own advocate. That's what I tell people when they're first diagnosed. Get on social media and find out what treatments are producing the best results and learn their side effects. I have a friend, Dr. Jack West, a top lung cancer specialist.

"'I treat patients all day long,'" he tells me, "'but you're out there researching every day. That's patient involvement.'"

"I think," Don says after our server steers away from our table yet again, "what Dr. West was also getting at is that I'm in a better position to scour the world for what's out there than maybe even he is. He's focused on hundreds of patients, while I'm only focused on one. I'll reach out to someone in my network who'll say something like, 'Hey, Don, I'm in this clinical trial for a very aggressive form of lung cancer and I've been cancer-free for over a year.' The problem is the FDA doesn't publish the results of the trial for over a year, so word might not get out to other patients who desperately need to know, and by then it may be too late to help them. But we make the results immediately available on Facebook. My group gets them first so the members can publicize them and put the results out there. I post everything about my journey on Facebook. I have a lot of brighter people then I am following me, and they'll call me out on something if they disagree. I share with them my firsthand experiences, and I know how much it helps. Helping is why I got involved in advocacy twenty-four/seven."

That's how he met the second love of his life (he and the mother of his children divorced after twenty years) in Penny Blume, a stage IV survivor of small cell lung cancer. They met on the internet on a cancer site called Inspire, a far cry from eHarmony or Match.com.

"We lived on opposite sides of the country, different coasts. We had talked and emailed regularly and she told me, 'All I'm looking forward to is making it to my fiftieth birthday.' I told her I'd buy her dinner, and she actually flew across the country to meet someone she'd never met to celebrate that occasion. A friend said to me that if I'd just met someone in a local Starbucks, she wouldn't have to fly three thousand miles so we could have a date. Penny's boyfriend had walked out on her as soon as she was diagnosed. He literally said, 'I didn't sign up for this.' I knew once we got involved I'd have to see this through to the end, and I was fine with that."

Don and Penny made sure to see each other every six weeks, rotating between their respective coasts until the fall of 2013, when Penny became too ill to travel. Don used as much vacation time as he could take or buy, and when that ran out, his boss allowed him to go out on disability to take care of her. He managed to sign Penny up for a clinical trial, but it was too late.

"I brought her to my home in California and cared for until her death on January 21, 2014. That was a really low point, the lowest of any I'd experienced since I'd been diagnosed. To think through all that I could get another chance at love, only to lose her. I took charge of her affairs, even emptied out her house after the funeral. We were soul mates in a way that's very difficult to describe. And I'd promised Penny shortly before she passed that I would continue to advocate for lung cancer awareness. Fulfilling that promise turned a low point into a high point, Penny affecting my life profoundly even after she was gone."

"You know," Don continues, after we give the waiter one final brush-off, "the last ten years of my life have been about the best. I tell people in the twelve-step program I'm in that I've got stage IV lung cancer and I wouldn't change places with anyone in this room. I've formed some of the most positive, inspiring relationships I've ever had, and the years I had with Penny were wonderful. When you have terminal lung cancer, you don't have to worry about who put the toilet paper roll on the wrong way. The fact that we couldn't be together all the time made our relationship stronger. We'd literally count down the days until we'd be seeing each other again, like a couple of kids."

We finally give the waiter a break and order our meals. I wonder what people might have been thinking, looking at the two of us huddled close, talking nonstop, in a steak house known for attracting the true power brokers of Capitol Hill. And here we were, a couple of lung cancer survivors.

Don and I make small talk until our appetizer arrives, the house Caesar salad already divided among two plates.

"My friend Matt would always say the easiest way to get through your hardest of times is to help someone through their hard times," he says, picking up where he left off. "I've become a fierce patient advocate for a number of lung cancer groups, and I'm a consumer reviewer for the Department of Defense Lung Cancer Research Program. I want to make sure no cancer survivor feels isolated and that all survivors have the information they need to become active participants in their own care."

I think about all the people Don has been there for and ask him who's been there for him through all his stages, the progressions, the maddening stops and starts that so typify lung cancer treatment, which requires substituting one drug for another whenever the one you're on loses its effectiveness.

"My one go-to person I've had since the day I was diagnosed is my friend Tim. We're in the same twelve-step group, and I've been his sponsor for twenty-five years. He drove me to the appointment when I was first diagnosed and has been there for me every step of the way—even up to a month ago, when I became anemic because of the current treatment I'm on. I was too weak to even walk from the bedroom to the living room, so he moved in to take care of me, helped me get to appointments. What I've learned from being in a twelve-step program, and from mentoring inmates with drug and alcohol problems, is that you can't keep what you don't give away. I can't survive if I'm not willing to share what I know.

"I've got a friend from the cancer community going into hospice every week. People ask me how can I keep doing it. And the answer's simple: it's because I know I've given them hope. Anytime a patient calls me I try to leave them with a little more hope than they had when I answered the phone. People look at lung cancer as a death sentence when it really isn't. I mountain biked for four years after my diagnosis. There's this picnic table at the top of a mountain I was riding up with my friend who said, 'Man, I'd love to get there today.' So I said, 'I'm going to get there first.' And I did. I beat him up the mountain, and another friend who lagged behind us said, 'Don's got stage IV lung cancer and you couldn't beat him to the top.'"

But Don's treatment has seen its share of ups and downs, those maddening fits and starts. The treatment you're on is working and you feel great, until the day it doesn't and you don't anymore. He expands on that notion as we finish off our salads.

"The side effects can sometimes be more serious than the cancer itself, and you never know when they're going to hit. There was that time I could hardly breathe and, remember, Bonnie, you insisted I go to my oncologist to get checked out. It turned out I had three liters of fluid built up in my pericardial sac. The doctors drained it, but reporting such symptoms becomes like a catch-twenty-two because the doctors might end up pulling me off the current treatment that's saving my life. That's why a lot of cancer patients don't want to tell the truth of what's going on with them, out of that fear. But they need to because that's the only way pharmaceutical companies can make the drugs better. One of the great myths is that these companies have no souls and no hearts, when nothing could be further from the truth. They're dedicated, amazing people, and many of them are friends of mine. I even spoke in Chicago on the tenth anniversary of a drug that saved my life being approved. Thousands of people got to celebrate more birthdays because of that drug."

I ask Don if he recalls how we met.

"Sure, I was involved in that organization called LUNGevity at the time. They were doing great things, but I found myself missing that one-on-one contact and connection. That's when I met an ex-NFL football player named Chris Draft who'd lost his wife to lung cancer at the age of thirty-eight. She was a cheerleader and an attorney, and Chris went all over the country to spread the word that lung cancer could happen to anyone. You could be sitting next to someone in a stadium who had it. It was Chris who told me about the work your foundation was doing, and one Tuesday I showed up at one of your Living Room programs."

"I remember," I tell him as our server places our main courses down before us. "And I remember your story too."

There was only one targeted therapy at the time of Don's original diagnosis. His doctors had no idea whether it would work on him, but his oncologist let him give it a try and, miraculously, it did.

"When I first got diagnosed," Don says, "my first thought was I might not be able to beat this, but I'm going to give it a run for its money. I think it's vital to do your research, to know the next therapy that's coming if your next scan shows recurrence. That way you're prepared and your first thought isn't *Poor me*, it's *When can I start on the new drug?* So it helps to already know going in what that new drug is going to be. I've lived a full life. I don't feel like I've been cheated out of anything. A lot of the reason why I document my whole journey on Facebook is to help others get through theirs. In the meantime, I'm living the best life I can while pondering plan C to stay one step ahead of this disease mentally."

Don is keenly aware there's a very good chance his cancer will reoccur someday, and he intends to be ready when that day comes. He looks great, but he's been hospitalized three times in the past two years in the ICU

"Today, at sixty-four, I can look back on my life with satisfaction and a sense of accomplishment of a life well lived. I've raised wonderful children and have the love of family and friends. I still lead an active lifestyle and live every day to the fullest. But I don't take anything for granted. If it's my time, it's my time. What motivates, what keeps me going, is that every time I get a text or email, I can help somebody else. But I'm also aware when I can't do it. I need to take care of my own health, help myself, because if I don't, I won't be here to help anybody else."

In between bites, I ask him something I've been asking a lot of people who are heavily involved and vested in the lung cancer community.

"Give me your three wishes for the future."

Don rattles off his choices with nary a pause. "That lung cancer will become a chronic illness and not a terminal disease. That lung cancer will get its fair share of funding compared to other cancers. And that everybody who gets lung cancer has somebody they can reach out to who can give them hope."

Author's Note: Don finally lost his brave battle with lung cancer in the spring of 2020. We thought it was important to leave his chapter in this book as both a testament to a great man and a reminder of the realities of this awful disease.

A CONVERSATION WITH RAFFAELLA SORDELLA

Raffaella Sordella is an associate professor at the Cold Spring Harbor Laboratory, located in Cold Spring Harbor, New York. Two challenges in cancer biology guide her work: first, how tumors become addicted to certain gene products, and second, how tumors develop resistance to anticancer drugs. She's also a cancer survivor herself, her pancreatic cancer having been discovered early enough to be surgically removed.

Could you describe the basics of your work?

It starts with my work with the EGFR mutation, a truly groundbreaking discovery in lung cancer research. We were able to treat lung cancer patients with a specific genetic mutation, achieving remarkable results to the point where in some responses the tumor was pretty much gone after only six weeks. After nine months, though, virtually all the patients relapsed; their tumors came back. It became clear we needed a mechanism to deal with the resistance that was preventing the drug from binding to its target. Currently, our approach is to treat lung cancer with a first-line drug until it fails and then proceed to second-, third-, and fourth-generation drugs targeting that secondary mutation. So our focus now is trained on coming up with a mechanism, a bullet, that could eliminate resistance. That would make cancer treatment more like HIV, far more efficacious.

The reason why this is important is that research has found that tumors are highly heterogeneous, consisting of multiple types of cells. We have to treat all of those cells, all elements of the tumor from the beginning, because that's what contributes to the resistance. It's not the tumor that kills patients, it's the mutation. And if we can prevent the mutation, we can change the face of lung cancer, and all cancer, forever.

What do you enjoy most about the clinical side in the fight against cancer?

Those eureka moments that come after you've confirmed a hypothesis and realize that you're onto something that might be truly groundbreaking. One stage IV patient who benefitted from our research, for example, recently climbed Mount Everest. Oncologists deal directly with patients and see the effects of our work on people. Clinical researchers may not share that direct contact from the lab bench, but knowing your discovery can make an impact on thousands of people has been the most rewarding experience of my career.

What keeps you excited about your work?

Seeing the effects on real people, knowing that my work is consequential. To know that you can make a difference. In essence, what we're doing in my lab is trying to understand the mechanism of resistance in tumors that stops our treatments from working, intrinsic to lung cancer but hopefully applicable to other cancers as well.

But there's also a human side in play here, a shrinking gap between science and society that helps remind scientists how their work is affecting the greater society at large. I feel we have a moral obligation as researchers to engage patients and make the world aware of all the progress being made. There's a wonderful program called Swim Across America, for example, where researchers have the opportunity to meet the patients being treated with the drugs we created. And seeing how much people rely on us inspires us to keep doing what we're doing.

What is the biggest challenge involved in your research?

Losing patients because maybe you didn't do enough. But those moments of discouragement serve as motivation to do even more. It's easy to keep in mind what we're doing, but we can never let ourselves forget who we're doing it for.

What we really need to do, though, is move faster between the lab and the frontline oncologists who are treating the disease. These oncologists are great doctors but don't necessarily understand the science behind the drugs they're prescribing. On the other hand, we're not always informed on the complexities of the actual disease. That means speeding up translation from the lab bench side to the clinical side, and that kind of interaction is becoming more and more common in the world of lung cancer treatment. We're learning what it's like to be oncologists, and they're learning the language of molecular biology.

Peer into your crystal ball and tell me what lung cancer patients have to look forward to in the near and slightly more distant future.

Since 2004, lung cancer has become the most exciting cancer to research because of the understanding of the disease on the genetic and molecular levels. Lung cancer, in that respect, has become the poster child for new approaches to treating cancer. And for the future I see us finding the Holy Grail of treating lung cancer and all cancers: that being the successful deployment of smart drugs clinically developed to manage resistance. Do that and we'd be able to successfully treat 70 percent of all lung cancer patients, and that's what we're working on now. Do that and other treatments will follow, because a principle you can apply to one type of tumor can be applied to others.

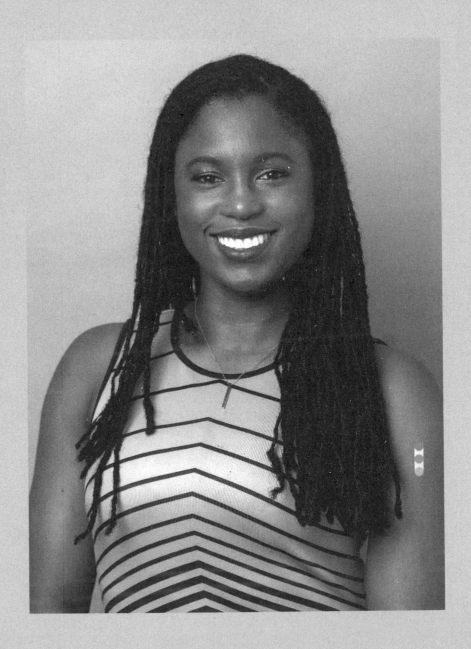

5

Sydney Barned, MD

What I also know is that you are stronger than you think. You will find an inner strength that you never knew you had. You will cry, and it's okay to shed those tears, but you will wipe your face and smile because you know you have no choice. You will look to your goals as your escape. You will use your experience as a patient to make you a better doctor. You will bring light to people who are in despair, because you will give them hope. You will inspire others around you and you will realize that your despair is short-lived because it could have been worse.

That's from a letter Dr. Sydney Barned wrote to herself shortly after being diagnosed with stage IV lung cancer at the age of thirty-three We've never met, but Laurie Fenton Ambrose, my partner in the merger that combined the Bonnie J. Addario Lung Cancer Foundation with the Lung Cancer Alliance in early 2019, told me I had to include her in this book.

Mere minutes into our phone conversation I could tell why.

"So I have to tell you what I was like when I was a kid," Sydney said, her voice carrying the slightest of accent from her native Jamaica. "According to my mom, I've always been active, even in utero when she could feel me kicking her ribs. As a toddler after watching the Olympics I started doing flips right there in the living room. My mom signed me up for a whole bunch of things to curb my energy: ballet, swimming, track, piano lessons. She always kept me busy. I've always been active, on the go. But one day I was jogging on the treadmill and started huffing and puffing like an old person. I ignored it because I wasn't old and figured I was just out of shape because say I had slacked off on my gym routine and hadn't been going as much as I used to.

"Turned out I was wrong."

Sydney speaks matter-of-factly, delivering this news to me in the processed tone of the doctor that she is, specializing in internal medicine currently at Howard University Hospital in Washington, DC. She's telling me about the weeks and months leading up to her initial diagnosis in February of 2017.

"A medical residency is all-consuming. Eighty-hour weeks that never seem to end, but I was loving it. Then, one weekend when I wasn't working in the emergency department of the University Hospital in Jamaica, I woke up feeling very tight on the left side of my chest. As a doctor, I knew the left lung wasn't getting enough air. So when I went into the hospital the next day, I made sure to get an X-ray."

The left side of her lung, Sydney recalls, was completely white. The radiology resident, who was also a friend, called upstairs and Sydney went up almost immediately to see doctors specializing in pulmonology who'd already viewed her X-ray before she got there.

"I told them about that experience on the treadmill, how I got short of breath all of a sudden and about the feeling I'd had in my chest when I woke up the day before. They asked me about weight loss, night sweats, any other examples of shortness of breath upon exertion. I told them no to all but that I'd been taking low doses of prednisone for about a year because of my eczema. They were convinced it must be pneumonia and put me on an antibiotic. I can't tell you why, but as soon as I started taking it, my symptoms worsened, starting with a spasmatic cough I couldn't control. I went to a top pulmonologist, who looked at my first X-ray and prescribed more steroids. He told me to repeat the X-ray in two weeks. But the consolidation—that's what it's called—was still there on the left side. The steroids should have cleared it but didn't."

A CT scan finally revealed a 3.5-centimeter mass that was compressing Sydney's airway.

"I freaked out, but at the same time I didn't think lung cancer, not right away. I must admit that I automatically linked lung cancer to smoking and, since I never smoked, it couldn't be lung cancer, right? I used to break my father's cigarettes in half so he couldn't smoke. I never actually saw him light up because he only smoked socially in a bar with his friends when he was drinking. I was obnoxious about cigarettes; I'd even tell my friends you can't smoke anywhere near me. I don't want to be exposed to those cancer sticks, I told them."

Then a bronchoscopy, a procedure that allows a doctor to examine the inside of the lungs, revealed the painful truth.

"The tumor was a highly vascular mass that bled when the pulmonologist touched it, a clear sign of cancer. Then a biopsy confirmed it, but found I was only stage I. Then a repeat test at Johns Hopkins found a lymph node that tested positive. That bumped me up to stage III. Hopkins also found cancer cells on the lining of my lungs, which meant I was elevated to stage IV. So within the span of the month, I went from being fine to having stage IV lung cancer."

The good news for Sydney, as for many lung cancer patients, was that biomarker testing revealed she was ALK positive, which made her a candidate for a targeted therapy that was a protein kinase inhibitor. Also like many lung cancer patients, that also meant she was able to avoid chemotherapy and all its side effects. That was two years ago.

"I just had a scan last month. Everything was clear, no evidence of disease anywhere."

The roller-coaster ride of lung cancer diagnosis and treatment, any cancer really, is impossible to describe. Only those who've lived through it can truly grasp it, and no two people or patients are alike. But what Sydney personifies perfectly is that lung cancer is a disease you no longer have to die of and can live with. The biomarker testing that didn't exist much more than a decade ago saved her life, and the targeted therapy is still working, doing its job just as Sydney continues to do hers at Howard University Hospital.

When first diagnosed, though, Sydney didn't know much more about lung cancer than the typical patient.

"I thought, *Well, crap. Well, damn. I wasted my whole life to go after this dream of being doctor and now I'm never going to do it. I should have traveled the world, become a hobo or something.* But one thing I did know about were the statistics, that only fifteen percent of lung cancer patients are alive after five years. It's hard to be optimistic in the face of something like that. You have to be realistic."

You could have found out that the cancer had spread to your brain. You could have found out that it had spread in your bones and you faced unbearable pain. You could have found out that you did not have a gene mutation and that you would have to do chemotherapy. You could have found out that you would have had to put your dreams on hold, possibly indefinitely. You could have found out that your love did not see a future with you because cancer was never in his plans. You could have not had the support you had. You could have all those, but you didn't.

At the end of each of the emails I received from Sydney in setting up this call, I noticed this quote: "Many extraordinary things are done by ordinary people who persevere!" Those words have become her credo, her life motto, and they've come to define a fight she has every intention of winning but knows she'll need to keep fighting for the rest of her life at this point.

"What that motto means to me is that you don't need to be super-duper brilliant, but what you need is to be super hard working and willing to push. But most important, you've got to be able to get up after you fall. You fall one time, you get up. You fall two times, you get up. You fall three times, you get up. There's a lot of things that aren't going to go your way all of the time, and you need resilience to get you back on the road where you need to be. The first time I applied to a residency program, I didn't get accepted, and that was the only way I could become a doctor in the States. My application wasn't good enough, so I came to the States and shadowed doctors for two months and got them to write letters of recommendation, and I got into a residency program on the second try. You need to see things through. Take little steps and then build upon those steps to get somewhere extraordinary."

Of course, some would say that surviving stage IV lung cancer for two-plus years is extraordinary in its own right. I ask Sydney what she'd tell a patient of hers if she learned they had lung cancer.

"I would tell them their life isn't over, that the chapter isn't closed and the book isn't finished. I'd tell them that a lot of it has to do with perspective and attitude. I'd tell them I've had stage IV lung cancer for two and a half years and I'm still here. That I completed my residency, working eighty hours per week, with cancer. I didn't even take a break from work, because I needed to work to remind me why I needed to fight so hard, because I wanted to practice medicine so badly. I think that for me having a positive attitude definitely helped, and I'd tell my patient there are so many innovations in treatment that are so positive we should all feel good about the direction things are going in."

I've known several medical professionals, including a wonderful doctor in the San Francisco Bay Area, who suffered from lung cancer themselves, but I never had the chance to ask any of them whether being a doctor is a hindrance or a help in dealing with the diagnosis.

"It's a bad thing initially because as a doctor I knew all too well that lung cancer has a very poor prognosis—that was the first thing that struck me. Numbers don't lie, so you can't be extremely optimistic, but they don't tell the whole story either. I had my whole life ahead of me. I'd found a guy, David, I wanted to be with. I wanted to have kids, buy a house. I'd worked so hard to become a doctor and now I was going to be dead in five years? As a doctor I saw the cold, hard realism of that. As a patient you can say I can beat this, I can be one of the lucky ones. But as a doctor I'd seen people who never get to be one of the lucky ones.

"Things had to change. I decided to keep my focus on internal medicine because I couldn't imagine changing my specialty and spending an additional three years of eighty-hour weeks. I want to be living my life. My whole perspective changed, and right around that time I went from the dark place of being one of the eighty-five percent to knowing I was going to be one of the fifteen."

I tell Sydney about my own dark moments and doubts, but I also ask about hers. Put two lung cancer survivors in a room (or on the phone!) and you've got an instant community. The bond we share has already broken down all barriers.

"Well," she tells me, "I always wanted to have kids so I could be the kind of mother to them my mother has been to me. But I can't have kids anymore, even though I had my eggs frozen. I know I'd still enjoy being a parent and it's just another challenge I have to get around."

On the other hand, Sydney has found that she's been able to have an emotional, almost visceral impact on the cancer patients who cross her path in the hospital in a way few other doctors can.

"I was on duty the day a breast cancer patient came in. She was despondent, ready to give up. I took her history and could see how down she was. So I said, 'Here's something I can tell you about myself to make you feel better.' I told her and she started looking at me in an entirely different way."

"'At the end of the day,' I said, 'I have stage IV lung cancer, but it could have been worse. It could be in my liver, my brain or bones. I might not be able to work.' I asked her, 'Is the cancer in your liver?'"

"'No,' she said."

"'Is it in your brain?'"

"'No.'"

"'Is it in your bones?'"

"'No.'"

"'How many treatments do you have left?'"

"'Two.'"

"And I could tell she felt better and left the hospital with a whole new attitude. A regular doctor couldn't have done that for her."

Sydney married her boyfriend, David, a month after her initial diagnosis. She tells me he's been there for her every step of the way. He goes to all of her appointments with her, every single scan. Initially, her mother, father, and sister took turns staying with her, but David is the only constant. Friends from Jamaica and Washington, DC, meanwhile, rallied at every turn, including two friends from her residency who started a GoFundMe page.

"I told them not to, but they did it anyway. It all just blew up on social media. I started hearing from people I'd gone to elementary school with in Jamaica and hadn't seen in twenty-five years."

That helped her through the initial diagnosis and treatment, along with never missing a beat on the requirements of her residency. Sydney loves what she does, loves being a doctor, and isn't about to let cancer get in the way of her dream. Still, it's a different dream now or, at least, a modified one.

"So many of my friends are buying homes right out of residency. As doctors, they can use their projected income to qualify for a mortgage. But I can't do that because if something should happen and God forbid I can't work anymore, I'd never be able to afford the house. David and I just moved into a new rental, and we're determined to save enough money to put down a substantial down payment on a house to take the pressure off. It all comes down to being very practical. I can't be cavalier about my income because I don't know if I'm going to still have it five or ten years from now. So while friends start to plan for retirement, I have to plan for what happens if I get sick."

She pauses over the phone for so long I think maybe I've lost the connection. Then her voice returns, unchanged.

"David always tells me I'm stronger than I think I am. He's also told me that one of the things he loves about me is how practical I can be.

How I'm able to remove emotion and see what needs to be done. He says that I inspire him, that when he gets frustrated with his work [as a graphic artist in the advertising field], he'll look at me studying or working and he'll think that I could have crawled into a corner but didn't."

Sydney is becoming more and more of a lung cancer advocate and credits advocacy groups in general with changing the very nature of how lung cancer is perceived and treated. That it no longer carries a death sentence and never really was strictly a smoker's cancer.

"Exploding that myth is vital. We've come a long way but still have a long way to go. When people think of a woman getting cancer, they think breast. With a man, it's colon or prostate. You see people living with other cancers in front of you, but until recently you didn't see survivors of lung cancer. Advocacy has changed all that, changed how people think of lung cancer. It needs to be understood, accepted, and treated the same way as other cancers and get the funding it deserves."

Sydney stops there, and I wait for her to continue. There's no reason to pose another question because I know she's going to answer whatever I have to ask on her own.

"I always come back to the Serenity Prayer, that God gave me the strength to accept the things I can't change and change the things I can, along with the wisdom to know the difference. I can't change my diagnosis, but I can change how I react to it. And it's made me a better doctor because my patients see that I'm human too, because I'm a doctor *and* a patient—I bridge that gap. I tell them you have to do this to save your life, because here's what I've done to save mine. Every day my phone alarm sounds twice to remind me to take my pills. That's a small price to pay for staying alive."

You will continue to see the true nature of your friends and family, that they love you and they will continue to rally around you. They will lift you up when you are stumbling and they will encourage you when you think that you can't continue. You will make it through residency, and walk across the stage. You remember your life quote and live up to it.

Here's an article I wrote in May of 2018 that has stuck with me ever since and I think will stick with you too. Meet the Ross-Wonders, cancer's new superheroes!

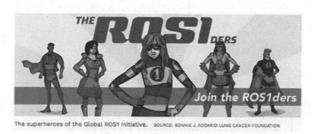

The superheroes of the Global ROS1 Initiative.   SOURCE: BONNIE J. ADDARIO LUNG CANCER FOUNDATION

You've likely never heard the story of how three young women, who call themselves "ROS1ders" from a rare form of lung cancer they share, may be turning the nation's 46-year-old war on cancer on its head. The women were diagnosed with a gene mutation called a ROS1 fusion. Less than 2 percent of lung cancer patients have that trait. They soon found out there was little research being conducted because of the difficulty in finding and collecting tissue samples. In other words, they were stuck with existing treatments and a drug designed for other types of lung cancers. Their future did not look bright.

"So we hatched a plan," Lisa Goldman, a mom in Silicon Valley trained as a lawyer, told me. Goldman, with Janet Freeman-Daily in Seattle, Washington, and Tori Tomalia in Ann Arbor, Michigan, asked a simple question: What if they could find other people around the world with ROS1-positive mutations who were willing to provide tissue samples to make a study feasible? Like many in today's hyper-connected digital world, they would use technology to hunt for patients regardless of location. They created a Facebook page, built a website, blogged, exploited social media, networked endlessly at conferences, and agreed on organizing principles. And they dubbed themselves—the ROS1ders (pronounced Ross-wonders).

In our celebrity culture, these ladies are not showy or impulsive. (Though their website has a flashy but cool video of them as cartoon superheroes!) If anything, they have courage, boldness, and the guts to face down the oftentimes smothering orthodoxy of cancer research.

One thing we know from experience is that most clinical trials fail because they don't have enough patients and the right amount of tissue samples. The ROS1ders took care of that. As of this writing, Lisa Goldman and her peers have located more than 200 ROS1ders.

"This is amazing for a lot of reasons," said Dr. Christine Lovly, MD, PhD, a noted cancer expert at the Vanderbilt University Medical Center. "In this case, it was the patients themselves who organized as a group" to launch a ROS1 study. "As far as I know it's the first time that's happened."

This patient driven, advocacy approach may prove to be a hugely important disruptive force for progress in how cancer research can be conducted quicker and more efficiently. There is not a lot of mystery about the ROS1der's motives. Like many cancer patients, they are facing death because research is lacking or not moving fast enough.

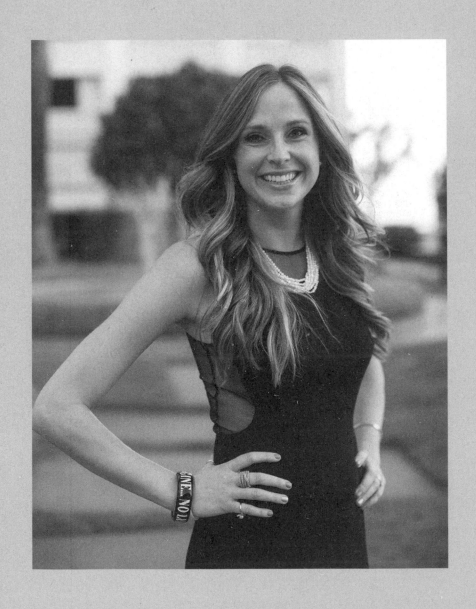

6

Emily Bennett Taylor

The cover of the September 26, 2016, issue of *Cancer Today* features a picture of a smiling Emily Bennett in the company of her then twin five-month-old daughters. She couldn't look happier or more beautiful, no inkling at all that just four years before she'd been diagnosed with lung cancer at the age of twenty-eight. In fact, when I told her I wanted to include her in this book, we had to schedule our conversations for when the now toddlers were napping.

We got lucky. They drifted off only five minutes after our scheduled start time. I could picture Emily racing into a separate room, baby monitor in hand, to call me back.

"Sorry about that," she says.

Emily tells me she's feeling great now nearly nine years since her lung cancer diagnosis. And almost since that day—June 28, 2012—she's been remarkably public about her experience. While many, if not most cancer patients prefer to endure their treatment in private, Emily decided to put hers out there for all to see.

"It started with my husband, Miles, going online and finding one story of hope to share with me every day to keep me going. That was quite a challenge, because he quickly realized there were next to none of them out there back then. No one was sharing their stories of cancer, particularly lung cancer, and that meant there wasn't enough hope out there. So I decided to chronicle my story as it unfolded. I believed so strongly that I would survive, I wanted other people to know that they could too. Just like me, they're going up against this great beast, and sharing my journey was all about letting them know they could fight and win. Sure, enduring chemotherapy is hard, but I wanted them to know how I made the chemo my ally because it was getting the cancer out of me. I'd close my eyes during my infusions and picture the drugs attacking cancer cells."

What's another of Emily's top recommendations for someone recently diagnosed with lung or any cancer?

"Having caregivers in your life is crucial. Miles is my everything. We started dating in our early twenties and never stopped. I think I knew he was the one from the first time we met. The strange thing was he was always the hypochondriac and it was me that got sick. He did everything he could to keep me positive. Long after I went to sleep, he'd be up researching and reading everything he could find out there on lung cancer treatments, even scientific journals. He was going to find a solution. It's so important to have someone like that; someone to drive you to appointments, steer you through those times that feel hopeless, be your champion and your advocate. Our life was lung cancer. We put everything else on hold, including having kids, because we had no choice."

"Patients need to find a support system," she continues, "like your GO2 Foundation. There's no reason to go it alone when you've got so many people out there who've been there and done that. And I thought if I shared my story in real time, I could be part of that support system for others."

A persistent cough and some shortness of breath sent Emily to her primary care doctor in 2012. An X-ray was ordered that revealed some haziness in her right lung, but lung cancer? Emily was too young and healthy for that, right?

Wrong. A follow-up CT scan and biopsy revealed cancer in her right lung that had spread to the surrounding lung lining, meaning the cancer was stage IV. She didn't know it then, but at the time statistics showed that just 10 percent of people diagnosed with stage IV non-small cell lung cancer lived five years or longer.

"Miles never told me that," Emily elaborates. "It came up in the research he did, but he didn't want me to know. That's what makes for a great caretaker: somebody who knows what not to tell you too!"

"Those days are crystal clear to me," she continues after a pause. "When I was on the elliptical machine, I'd breathe in and feel a wheeze in my breath. It came and went. Several weeks later I was still exercising, still playing volleyball, but my coughing got more and more persistent. My doctor figured it was allergies or maybe asthma and prescribed an inhaler. That worked sometimes, but the cough kept getting worse. So I went to see a pulmonologist, who prescribed a chest X-ray. I was in his waiting room reading this pamphlet on lung cancer and I called Miles right away."

"'I've got all these symptoms of lung cancer,'" I told him.

"'You don't have lung cancer,' he told me."

"And, sure enough, the pulmonologist diagnosed me with asthma. She said I could still get a chest X-ray if I wanted, and I was actually halfway out the door when I went back inside to get one. The pulmonologist read it immediately and noted that the entire right lung was covered in this hazy fog."

"'What does that mean?'" I asked her.

"'I've seen thousands of patients,'" she said. "'And no one young and healthy like you gets lung cancer.'"

"But, to be on the safe side, she ordered follow-up with a CT scan. The next day I got a call at work from her telling me to come in. One thing I've learned is that it's never good news when the doctor asks you to come in. I was the only one in her office when I got there.

"But her initial diagnosis wasn't lung cancer; it was lymphoma. Because, again, nobody young and healthy gets lung cancer. She ordered a biopsy which proved otherwise."

I first met Emily in September of 2012, shortly after her diagnosis when she came to San Francisco to participate in a 5K run and walk my foundation was sponsoring. To say we hit it off immediately would be an understatement, and I got the sense that was true for just about anyone who gets to meet Emily. She brightens any room she enters, looking trim, athletic, and fit with a smile stretched from ear to ear. It was a lot harder, though, for her to smile back then, when her future was still uncertain and she was beginning a journey that would define whether she and Miles would have a future.

Thanks to brave women like Emily, and to better understand the special traits of lung cancer in young adults, the Addario Lung Cancer Medical Institute, our partner nonprofit that represents an international consortium of more than twenty-five research organizations, embarked on the Genomics of Young Lung Cancer study. Our goal was to look at the adolescent/young adult population (AYA), people under forty who've been diagnosed with non-small cell and small cell lung cancer.

That might not seem like a big deal, but until women like Emily Bennett and others came forward, lung cancer was perceived to be an older person's and a smoker's disease. And we can't help all the Emilys out there until we take a wrecking ball to these mythologies that for so long have permeated both medicine and pop culture. Think about that for a moment. Think about the fact that Emily's twin girls, Hope and Maggie, who were napping at that moment, never would have been born if she hadn't gone back into that doctor's office to get a chest X-ray she'd just been told she didn't need.

Because she was young.

Because she never smoked.

I wish I was in that room to give Emily a big hug to thank her for all the lives her story was helping to save by driving awareness and educating other young women on the real demographics of lung cancer.

Everyone wants to believe it can't happen to them, until it does. As I form that thought, I can hear a sound over the phone coming out from the baby monitor, one of her girls cooing in her sleep. I wait for it to stop and ask Emily to talk about the most important messages she'd like people to take from her story.

"Well, I think you have to believe that although the odds may not be great, that the deck may be stacked against you, there are survivors and you will be one of them. It's okay to be sad sometimes, let yourself heal, pick yourself up and keep fighting. You get told you're only going to have one lung, and you get a scan result that's stable and start worrying about the next scan right away. You worry about what you'll do when the treatment's not working anymore. Someone sent me a refrigerator magnet I look at every day: 'When you're going through hell, keep going.' I don't know why that's stuck with me, but it has. I guess because it alludes to the fact that there's a light at the end of the tunnel, and if you keep going, you'll get there. Having lung cancer feels like you're in the middle of a hurricane with no eye, no calm amidst the storm, but if you keep fighting, you'll get to the other side."

For Emily, and Miles, that other side is the twin girls currently napping in another room. Having a family remained their overriding goal, one they wouldn't let be waylaid by her cancer. So before starting chemotherapy, Emily's eggs were harvested and fertilized in a process called in vitro fertilization. Within three weeks of her diagnosis, the couple had nine frozen embryos stored for later use. Then they turned all their energy to Emily's cancer treatment, though not exactly as originally prescribed. Emily, and Miles again, relentlessly insisted on surgery to remove the side of her lungs where the cancer had originally taken root. Even though the chemo treatments had been successful in shrinking the tumor dramatically, surgery seemed by all accounts to be the surest way of avoiding recurrence. The problem was surgery is almost always a nonstarter for stage IV lung cancer patients. Emily and Miles, though, were not to be denied.

91

Emily and her family asked friends and advocacy organizations for the names of surgeons with experience who might be willing to perform the risky operation. After four surgeons said no, Dr. Raja Flores, chairman of the thoracic surgery department at the Icahn School of Medicine at Mount Sinai in New York City, said he'd consider it.

"You can get many surgeons who wouldn't agree with doing this procedure," Flores told *Cancer Today* for Emily's 2016 cover story. "This is definitely pushing the envelope, and if I did not see that fight in Emily, I would not have done the surgery, because it takes a lot to get through."

But he still didn't definitively agree to perform surgery, not until Emily's scans confirmed the tumor was isolated. "In early February [of 2013]," the *Cancer Today* cover story continues, "Flores did video-assisted thoracic surgery to confirm that the cancer was in the lung's lining. After confirmation, he performed an extrapleural pneumonectomy, removing Emily's diseased right lung, the linings of the chest cavity and lung, a portion of her diaphragm, and lymph nodes. He also removed and rebuilt the membrane surrounding her heart. After surgery, Flores told the couple he was confident he had removed all the cancer he could see. Two days later, the couple posted to their blog a video of Emily in the hospital slowly dancing down the hall while steadying herself with her walker."

Again, sharing her story with the world in the hope it would save more lives.

But Emily wasn't out of the woods yet, far from it. She endured an agonizing twenty-eight rounds of high-dose radiation to kill the disease once and for all. She pictured the invisible radiological beams slaying the cancer, as she had with her initial doses of chemotherapy.

"Having been an athlete," she told *Cancer Today*, "I always felt that I could push myself and do anything I wanted to do, and that just got stripped away from me. That was really frustrating, but I didn't let it be a big focus in my life because I knew there were more important things to focus on."

And those important things turned out to be Hope and Maggie. Since I have two daughters myself, I could relate to what Emily wanted so desperately to experience. My adult daughters, and son, were all the motivation I needed to fight my cancer. Through the dehumanization and indignity of fighting to survive cancer, through the days where I couldn't get out of bed or, when I did, make it all the way to the bathroom in time, I found the strength I needed to persevere in my children. If I couldn't endure it all for myself, then I could endure it all for them. The difference with Emily, of course, was that she was persevering and enduring in pursuit of a pipe dream. Lung cancer survivors don't have children. They're too busy trying to live themselves.

"The key moment in the process for me came years before," she says. "And you'll remember it, because you were right there. You sent me a picture, like a poster, with SURVIVOR printed on it. I told you I was only four months into my treatment and maybe that wasn't right, like premature. But you were adamant. You said, 'No, you get to claim that title because you are a survivor. Claim that word because it defines your future and your present. Claim that word.' You said that twice, remember?"

I did, with crystal clarity. The vast majority of us have never had a friendship with someone who's been told they may not, probably won't, make it to see the next Christmas. What happens then is that everything in your life takes place with the camera on zoom, a kind of hyper-focus in which moments can feel like hours, hours like days, and days like months. And every one of those moments is meaningful and something to be cherished. I know what it's like for somebody to be fighting against the odds, because I'd been there. And you win by not believing for a single second that the disease is going to beat you. You win by acting like you've already beaten it.

But even for Emily, pregnancy was something else again.

Since research shows that lung cancer reoccurrence normally happens within two years, Emily and Miles pushed themselves to wait that long before starting a family. As things turned out, it took all of that for her to regain the strength and vitality so sapped by chemotherapy, radiation, and surgery.

Then they hit another snag.

"Doctors also advised Emily that carrying and delivering a baby might be too much for her body," Marci Landsmann writes in *Cancer Today*, "so in April 2015, she celebrated two years with no evidence of disease by updating the couple's blog with a call to anyone who might be willing to carry and give birth to the Taylors' baby."

The rest is a history, an incredibly pleasant one at that. Emily and Miles found their gestational surrogate and on April 20, 2016, their twin girls were born. An incredible triumph of persistence and bravery that serves as inspiration for lung cancer patients everywhere of what is possible.

Yes, it's true that Emily can't do everything she could before her cancer. She has limitations she's learned to live and cope with, never complaining or bemoaning what she can no longer do because she knows that she is a miracle and has twin girls to prove it.

"These days, Emily, now thirty-two," the *Cancer Today* cover story concludes, "spends a lot of time on the couch trying to get the babies to smile, a behavior they mastered at two months. She still works on overcoming lingering physical limitations. For example, getting up and down is difficult for her, so she keeps the babies on the couch, which is lined with a diaper caddy, television remotes, toys and anything else the new mom might need for herself or her little ones. Emily's parents, Kevin and Shelley Bennett, who live in Memphis, Tennessee, and Miles' parents, Michele and Rich Taylor, from Sacramento, California, stay with the couple for weeks at a time in their Woodland Hills, California, home to help care for the babies. In addition, when Maggy and Hope were infants, the couple had a night nurse five days a week to handle overnight feedings. The arrangement allowed Emily to get the ten to twelve hours of sleep a night she needs."

Emily's story encapsulates the tenets of lung cancer treatment and recovery: hope, determination, and persistence supplemented by a great caregiver support system and the best medical care available. And Emily's story also highlights that you won't be the same person you were before you got cancer and beat it as you will be after. Like her, you may emerge an even stronger person on the other side.

But that doesn't mean Emily hasn't experienced her share of dark moments where the abyss came calling.

"I'll tell you a story," Emily begins. "Three or four months into my treatment, I was starting to understand a little more about the odds I was facing that Miles had hid from me initially. I had gone through four or five rounds of chemo and I started to face the possibility that I wasn't going to be okay, that this wasn't going to end well. One night, Miles and I were watching a movie. I can't even remember the title but it was a sad movie where a character passes away at the end. We both lost it. Miles doesn't like sad movies to begin with, and I think everything just boiled over for the two of us in that moment. I was twenty-eight years old and shouldn't have to deal with my own mortality. It seemed so unfair that I might not be able to beat this. And that would be unfair for anyone, not just me. We all have to deal with our own mortality, but nobody should have to do it this way at twenty-eight."

That dark moment, to be forever held in memory, has made Emily appreciate all the more the fact that she's no longer in that "danger zone, not standing on the precipice." I can personally relate to that kind of emotional roller coaster ride that is part and parcel of lung cancer treatment. The key for survivors like Emily and me is to be grateful for and cognizant of the fact that the highs have come to outnumber the lows.

"My life has changed in a lot of physical ways," she says softly to me over the phone. "And I'm acutely aware of all it took to get here. The girls will be playing, or reach some milestone, or say something funny. And I laugh, thinking about seven years ago, and all it took to get here." I can picture her shaking her head on the other end of the line. "The things people take for granted.... Life happens and puts things in perspective. I'm calmer now when someone cuts me off on the road, or

I'm waiting on hold forever, or stuck in some line. I'm here, and that's all that matters. Whatever life throws at me now, I can handle it with appreciation for all that I have because I fought for it."

SURVIVOR PREVAILS OVER LUNG CANCER WITH PRECISION MEDICINE AND VOLUNTEERISM

Precision medicine has prolonged life for many with lung cancer, giving them opportunities to support those who are newly diagnosed.

By Beth Fand Incollingo
Published May 21, 2019, in *CURE* magazine

Paul Ehlin will never forget the doctor's crushing words to his wife, Audrey, when she was diagnosed with lung cancer: "We'll give you six months and keep you comfortable."

"That was 12 years ago," Paul, accompanied by Audrey, told a room full of lung cancer survivors, caregivers and their doctors at a meeting Fort Lauderdale, Fla., on May 16. "In the last couple of years, she'd do yearly scans, and every year they were good. She had a scan six months ago and they said, 'You've got cancer in your other lung.' But I now know that you have to have a lot of hope."

Prevailing over lung cancer with precision medicine—and by taking personal action to help stamp out the disease—were the themes of the meeting held by the GO2 Foundation for Lung Cancer, an organization formed by the recent merging of the Bonnie. J. Addario Lung Cancer Foundation and the Lung Cancer Alliance. Numerous patients and caregivers told stories of precision treatments—CyberKnife, targeted drugs and immunotherapy—that have allowed them to manage lung cancer as a chronic condition, meeting health challenges as they come up but continuing with the activities of their lives.

Given their improved overall prognosis, many survivors asked how they could give back to the lung cancer community, and the GO2 Foundation had answers: Use personal networks to encourage those eligible to undergo screening for lung cancer, share cancer journeys with legislators to help secure government funding for research, and find ways to offer emotional support to patients beginning their journeys.

"We never had advocates before, because nobody survived," said Dr. Luis E. Raez, chief of hematology/oncology and medical director at Memorial Cancer Institute in Fort Lauderdale, where all the patients who attended are treated. "Now, you guys are surviving, and hopefully some of you are cured, and that's why we have the opportunity to also make a difference for the new patients to come."

The meeting was one in a monthly series of Lung Cancer Living Room sessions that bring together doctors, nurses, patients, survivors and caregivers to discuss specific issues related to the disease. The sessions include personal stories, advice and support, clinical information and updates on leading-edge research. They occur across the country but are livestreamed on social media to reach everyone interested.

Raez moderated the May panel of health care providers that also included nurse navigator Mihaela Roldan; radiation oncologist Dr. Ana Botero; thoracic surgeon Dr. Francisco Tarrazzi; and medical oncologist Dr. Gelenis Domingo.

The practitioners called upon patients and their loved ones to take action in numerous ways.

Raising Money and Awareness

Raez suggested that patients collaborate with the GO2 Foundation to raise funds and awareness.

"More and more, we're seeing survivors, and if they talk and raise awareness, we'll have better results," he said. "It's a matter of changing your environment, your close network.… There are minor or major things we can do—every single person and every relative. We can create an impact."

The GO2 Foundation offers many suggested ways for those affected by lung cancer to help: launching fundraising campaigns or grassroots events, donating money, financially supporting an awareness or fundraising event, employee gift matching, volunteering in various small or big ways, or buying the organization's branded products.

Lobbying

Emily Eyres, the chief program officer for the GO2 Foundation, asked patients and their families to support the Women and Lung Cancer Research and Preventive Services Act of 2018, which would fund a national awareness campaign about lung cancer in women and the importance of prevention, and expand lung cancer screening to people who don't fit the current criteria.

"We need you to come to Washington in July when have our 11th Annual National Advocacy Summit and tell your stories to your legislative officials," she said. "Tell them to support this historic legislation. Your elected officials listen to you. We want to get every state representative to support this."

The summit will take place July 21 through 23 at the Washington Marriott at Metro Center in Washington, D.C. It will bring like-minded people together and train them to tell their stories to legislators, with whom meetings are pre-scheduled.

Offering Emotional Support

Patients and survivors interested in serving as "buddies" to people newly diagnosed with lung cancer have a couple of options, those at the meeting were told.

GO2 has a phone buddy program that has been in operation for nearly 20 years. It matches up similarly diagnosed patients and their caregivers based on gender, age and types of treatments and side effects. "A lot of the phone buddies have been involved the whole time, and many for a decade, if not longer," Eyres said.

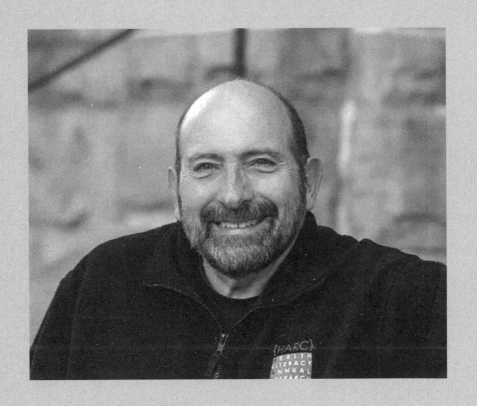

7

Jim Pantelas

My wife was six and a half months pregnant on the day I was diagnosed with stage 3B, non-small cell lung cancer. That was eleven years ago and I've been dancing with NED (no evidence of disease) for the past ten years. But dancing doesn't necessarily mean having fun.

Words from Jim Pantelas in a post for the Lung Cancer Alliance in April of 2017. I first met Jim in Washington at the National Lung Cancer Advocacy Summit, the purpose of which is to train our community's own activists (almost exclusively patients and caregivers) how best to approach their own congressional representatives and other politicians to advocate for more research dollars.

"I learned how to talk to congressmen here," he tells me. "I introduce myself as a thirteen-year survivor of lung cancer, but I also tell them how it breaks your heart to live in a community where we lose a friend every week and four hundred and thirty-two people in total per day, a fact that pretty much flies under society's radar. Then I'll ask what their lung cancer story is. It almost always turns out they have a friend or relative with the disease, so they can relate. Everything gets so much more personal and poignant when it's about them than when it's about me. I want it to be about their story, not mine, about someone they love who's dying or has died. If you have lungs, you can get lung cancer—that's the overriding point."

When we steal a few minutes to speak in a small sitting area off one of the conference rooms, our conversation darts back those thirteen years to when Jim was diagnosed and his wife was six and a half months pregnant with their first child.

"I had surgery where doctors took out most of my right lung. Because the cancer had metastasized, that was followed up by both radiation and chemotherapy treatments. Our daughter Stella was born the day of my second infusion."

Can you imagine? Life does pile on at times, but it wasn't done yet with the Pantelas family. Their newborn daughter, Stella, had been home for only five days when she suffered a brain bleed that resulted in her suffering seventeen seizures in the next twenty-one days.

"I spent most of my time in between my treatments at St. Joseph's Hospital going to Children's Hospital at the University of Michigan. That's when Stella was diagnosed with cerebral palsy that left her a quadriplegic."

I've heard the story before, but somehow hearing it again feels like the first time. It's like when you rewatch a movie that ends tragically hoping for a different outcome. But Jim doesn't consider himself the victim of tragedy or even any more courageous than anyone else.

"I don't think there's any courage involved. I had to live because I couldn't die. I think of life as a strange journey along parallel roads of science and faith. When you go through something like this, when the life you were expecting and planning for changes, you have to re-create yourself with new parameters. You get the opportunity to be resurrected."

Jim's analytical approach to the tragedies that came to define his life was born of an earlier career with the National Security Agency (NSA), where he worked on big data projects.

"I've been around big data all of my life, so I tend to think of life in terms of iterations. I have stepsons who are now in their mid-forties. How do I teach them how a man lives and dies—because that's the job of a parent? That's not an issue of courage, that's an issue of responsibility, just like taking care of my family was."

He isn't emotional when he speaks, but you can nonetheless hear the passion in his voice. I've always thought of life as a game of checkers, but Jim Pantelas is clearly playing chess.

"Lung cancer is a strange disease. People blame you for getting it because of the smoking stigma. It's strange when you think that, for all the great work that it's done, the American Cancer Society has perpetuated that myth by relentlessly associating smoking with lung cancer. More than anything, those warnings on cigarette packs have left society judging you a victim of an addiction you never had. I'm talking about the myth that lung cancer is a smoker's disease, when there are far more sufferers who contracted the disease from radon, asbestos, or other environmental factors. And there's a ton of people out there who never smoked who are getting diagnosed in their twenties, thirties, and forties, thanks to genetic mutations we're just starting to understand."

And Jim is putting his data analytics skills to good use in that regard.

"I do a lot of advocacy work, and some of that work revolves around reviewing and overseeing studies as part of an institutional review board at the University of Michigan. We jokingly have a saying in my family: Forever forward. You don't have an option. You either go forward or you die. You get out of bed in the morning and go forward, and if you get the chance, you do it again tomorrow. I don't fear death. I don't think death is the enemy. What happens when you die? You go back from whence you came. It's all about going home."

Jim was diagnosed after being sick for a year. He'd been running his own company for fifteen years, with offices in California and Michigan, where he makes his home. The company served as a recruitment process outsource, working with companies that were trying to grow but hadn't found the right people yet to position them for expansion. Those companies would outsource all their hiring to Jim.

"I was tired all the time and had to curtail my workload. Ultimately, I closed my California office in San Ramon, and with the reduced workload came a drop in income. When I got diagnosed, I had to think about how I was going to pay what were sure to be six- or even seven-figure medical bills, even with good health insurance. The problems that you think are important are still important when you get diagnosed. You just end up with additional shit to deal with, but the day-to-day stuff doesn't go away. You still have to deal with all the things you dealt with before. It's not that those things suddenly become unimportant, they just become secondary."

In addition to dealing with lung cancer, Jim found himself having to deal with a child who was going to need round-the-clock care for her entire life. I look at him in the soft chair adjacent to mine. Some people wear their feelings on their sleeve. Jim seems to me more the type who internalizes things, including his own pain. There's nothing wrong with that, and if I've learned anything about lung cancer patients over the past fifteen years, it's that all of us deal with what's happening in our own way. We find a way to cope, fighting to survive, because as a whole the thousands of lung cancer patients I've met over the years are the bravest, most inspirational lot I can ever imagine. No two are the same. And what's most unique about them is the coping mechanisms they develop to deal with their disease, even as they're forever fighting to beat it.

For Jim, that coping mechanism, more than anything, was volunteering.

"So what does a workaholic do with his life when he can no longer work?" he wrote in a post for the Lung Cancer Alliance in April of 2017. "He volunteers! I began volunteering ten years ago—first at the Children's Hospital that took care of my daughter, and then more and more in support of lung cancer funding, legislation and research. That involvement is now a major part of my life. I started with assignments to review multiple research proposals as a peer reviewer for PCORI (Patient Centered Outcomes Research Institute). I represented the non-scientist and patient perspective on an oncology IRB (Institutional Review Board) at the university where I volunteer. I also sat on an IRB for my local Veterans Administration Hospital, and I participated in two IRB meetings for the NCI (National Cancer Institute) where I'm also a regular board member. I followed up on two research efforts that I helped to develop and worked on a draft for a research project I want to pursue. I sat on a Pediatric Ethics Committee (and have for the past 10 years), chaired a Patient Experience Board, was a member of a Cancer Council and participated in a Quality Panel for the hospital where I receive my care."

Some might read that and believe Jim's doing it because he wants to escape, to find excuses to busy himself with something other than his daughter's chronic care and his own illness. He scoffs at the mere notion of that, finding it absurd.

"Why do I do all this? Mostly, I'd say, because it all matters. Maybe it's because I'm still alive and this is my way of paying back the universe for allowing me to continue breathing. But in reality, it's also because I love what I'm doing. The work I do has value to my lung cancer community and it has value to my family."

Something else I've noticed about the lung cancer community. The resilience of patients, the strength that comes from a part of them that's undefinable, is impossible to fathom. They don't see themselves as heroes, and it's never only themselves they're fighting this battle for, it's always for someone else too.

"I took care of myself from the outset," Jim says over the voices in the hall rising from those exiting the sessions that just ended, "because I didn't want any distractions from what Stella needed. Everything she and my wife needed came first, and maybe that's why, I tell people, that's why I've survived: because I didn't have to think about myself. I drove myself to every chemotherapy and radiation treatment. I didn't ask anyone to step up or in to help me, because I wanted the focus to be on them helping my family instead. There were times I was too weak to even walk up the stairs to the nursery to help my wife with Stella."

Jim may have spent his career in data analytics, a cause-and-effect guy, but he's also a great storyteller with a keen notion of the human condition and how the smallest gifts loom so much larger when received at the most opportune of times.

"It's real hard for cancer patients to ask for anything for themselves. On my Facebook page, I have a heart made out of sentences, out of words. Look closely and you'll see it's a primer for things you can do for someone that's suffering. The treatments for my cancer extended into the winter, and it happened to be a winter where we had a ton of snow in Michigan. But every time I came home, the driveway would be plowed and clear because a neighbor of mine took it on himself to do it. I got home from surgery to find another neighbor mowing my lawn. People who knew what I needed just did it, without being asked or prompted. I never asked them to do anything, but they did it anyway because that's the way people are when you give them a chance. These days, when I go and see someone who's sick with cancer, I'll buy a bunch of stuff for them I think that might taste good. I'll ask them how they're doing, if there's anything else they need. Then I leave, because I don't want them to feel like they need to use up their strength entertaining me."

Jim and I first met at the Lung Cancer Alliance summit two years ago. He recognized right away that the primary advocacy organizations for lung cancer aren't in competition with each other. We're all fighting the same battle, and it's a battle much better fought together, side by side and shoulder to shoulder. Otherwise, the patients are the ones who suffer. Jim got that, which led to the bond we formed. We didn't see ourselves as strangers or rivals but travelers on the same journey, making the same stops along the way.

Jim, after all, has plenty on his mind already, in addition to his lung cancer. Taking care of a special needs child with a myriad of challenges is something neither I, nor any other lung cancer patient I've met along the road of this journey, has experienced. But he isn't just up to the task; he's taken it on with the humility and commitment that defines his personality.

"We have an eye gaze machine on order that will allow Stella to communicate directly with us for the very first time," he tells me, truly excited by those prospects and for good reason. "It's going to be fairly rudimentary, pretty much just yes and no, but for Stella just to be able to say no would be huge for us."

The machines were designed primarily with ALS (a.k.a. Lou Gehrig's disease) patients in mind. These systems rely on eye movement to pick out various letters on a computer screen to allow the patient to form a word or entire message, requiring only the capacity to have upper and lower as well as lateral eye movement. Since Stella lacks the cognitive skills to manage more than basic communication, starting with yes or no will be a game changer for her, Jim, and the entire Pantelas family. But the strength and confidence he exudes belie the kind of thoughts that sometimes keep him, and virtually all lung cancer survivors, awake long into the night.

"What scares me? Damn near everything," he wrote me in a subsequent email. "I get a headache and the first thought is brain metastasizes. I still get 'scanziety' every year before my annual CT scan. And I'm dreadfully afraid that I'll live longer than my funds will hold up, and that I'll be worth more to my family dead than alive. I'm afraid that I'll not be around to see my girls graduate from junior high, let alone high school or college. And I'm afraid that someone else will end up being considered their dad by then. Mortality? Shit, I don't know. I'm sixty-six years old. My dad died (of small cell lung cancer) when he was sixty-seven years and forty days old, and his was a brutal passing. As I approach that age (less than a year away) I wonder if I'll live longer than he did. And I wonder if my name will pass anyone's lips a year or two after I'm gone. I do what I do because I want to try to make sure my girls don't ever have to deal with the disease that will have killed their father, and the grandfather they never knew."

In spite of those occasionally difficult times, Jim lives his life on an incredibly even keel. After all he's been through, nothing seems to roil or rattle on him, his approach and manner the polar opposite of someone whose shoulders break under the weight of life's piling on. When he talks about Stella, though, there's a different tone to his voice, coming straight from the heart.

"We were vacationing at Mackinac Island a few years back," he recalls, a reflective smile flashing thinly, "which is a small island, maybe eight miles around, tucked between two peninsulas of Michigan. Mackinac's claim to fame is that no cars are permitted. You get around by carriage, bicycle, or horseback. It was Fourth of July weekend, so the island was packed. I tell my wife, Kathy, that when we're on vacation, I take care of Stella so she and our other two daughters can go off and spend money. I was standing in the lobby of the Chippewa Hotel with Stella when this woman came me up and asked me if Stella was tube fed. She asked a bunch more questions, and it turned out she lived on the island and had a daughter named Olivia who'd passed away and reminded her of Stella. She told me that the carriages on the island are now outfitted with wheelchair lifts because of her advocating on her daughter's behalf.

"She also had a special bicycle made for Olivia that was basically a bike in the back, with an electric motor on the rear wheel, and a wheelchair in the front. She told me all about it. We were actually staying on the mainland, and the next day she called me and asked if I could be around the ferry stop for the boat's 2:15 arrival. I said I could and when the ferry arrived, she got off with the custom-made bike in tow, the very last thing she had of her daughter's. It hadn't been run in the six years since Olivia died, and she thought Stella was the perfect person to have it. I researched the bike when I got home; turned out it was manufactured in the Netherlands at a cost of around fifteen thousand dollars. I got it fixed up and it holds a charge for thirty miles. When summer rolls around, I take it over to Stella's school so the other kids can use and enjoy it too for those months. Teachers take pictures every year of kids getting a ride. You can tell how happy they are, how much the ability to experience something we would never think twice about changes their lives. And we send those pictures to Olivia's mom so she can see that her daughter's bike is being put to good use."

That's Jim. Unceasingly analytical, while always speaking from the heart, a unique combination for sure but one that has served him very well.

We both have sessions coming up and rise to make our way to our respective conference rooms. But not before Jim tells me about his other two kids. His nine-year-old daughter, Leda, is already an accomplished equestrian who rides American Saddlebred horses in competitive meets all over the country. And his eleven-year-old girl, Grace, dances competitively and is headed for the Nationals as I write this in 2019.

"These are the things," he says, "that get me out of bed in the morning."

The equestrian academy where Leda learned to ride, only four miles from their home, was actually founded by a woman who lost her son to cancer at the age of fifteen. Jim met her at the Michigan hospital where he does the bulk of his volunteering.

"It's all about community."

Jill Costello, whom you will meet in chapter 8, didn't survive her battle with lung cancer. And yet the bravery she displayed throughout her courageous struggle in which she refused to quit has offered hope and inspiration to countless other patients who hold her in an esteem worthy of the heroism she so brilliantly represents. Jill never gave up hope, something beautifully articulated in this post for Behind the Ink in November of 2014 by another "Jill" you'll meet later in these pages.

NEVER SAY NEVER: A PERMANENT REMINDER

Jill Feldman
—for my entire family; past present and future

Never say Never… Admit it; we have all declared at one time, in some way, "I will never…!" I know I have. There are many things I said I would never do that have been refuted, but one thing I said I would never, ever do, is get a tattoo. I didn't judge people who had them, but they weren't for me. Tattoos are a lifelong commitment and unlike bell-bottom pants and baggy sweaters, tattoos cannot simply be thrown in a giveaway pile and be forgotten about!

As we all know, life is all about change, and I've had some life-changing experiences that have led me to a change of heart about tattoos. In fact, one of the things I didn't like, the permanency of a tattoo, is what led me to getting one…actually, I got two tattoos ~ Go big or go home!

The first time I thought of getting a tattoo was five years ago, when I was diagnosed with lung cancer. I would casually mention it in conversation, but I wasn't committed and didn't even know what design I wanted to get. And then, not by choice, I got my first tattoos in May 2013. They are boring, ugly, and not what I would choose—they are tattoo-like markings for the radiation I had on one of the cancers in my lungs!

I am okay with the radiation tattoos, the scars I have from surgery and the marks left on my skin from a targeted therapy drug used to fight my lung cancer. I earned every one of them and wear them proudly, but they weren't my choice. Lung cancer, indirectly, created them. My defiant-self decided that the next marks on my body were going to be my choice; what I want and where I want. I was back to thinking about getting a tattoo.

Fast forward to last May. I was at LUNGevity's HOPE Summit in Washington DC where over 100 lung cancer survivors came together to learn, have fun, provide support and share hope. Hope is a word that I never used to associate with lung cancer because in my experience there was only false hope, or no hope at all. But as LUNGevity has grown and advancements in research have been benefitting patients more and more, I have started to believe that there is hope and I have started using the word more.

HOPE Summit 2014 really opened my eyes and my mind to hope, and it came at the perfect time. I was finally in a good place accepting that my Stage 1 lung cancer had evolved into a Stage 4a diagnosis. I looked around the room in awe as I listened to survivors tell their stories, I watched the interaction among survivors and caregivers, I heard about the latest advancements in research, I felt the virtual (and often real) hugs and I embraced the support—I experienced hope for the first time. Hope had a whole new meaning to me.

Hope is a powerful force. Hope means different things to different people at different points in their journey. The hope I saw transpire in that room was real. It wasn't about wishing for a miracle or dreaming of a cure. It was hope that lights the way during dark times. Hope that means being realistic but not giving up. Hope that means having faith and believing that nothing, even cancer, can defeat the human spirit. Hope that provides the strength to get up every morning and face each day. It may not sound like much, but after what we have all gone through, it is a lot—Hope is everything!

So, at Hope Summit I started thinking more seriously about getting a tattoo—a tattoo about hope. As long as I'm realistic, there is always hope, and I never wanted to forget that feeling. A tattoo that simply said hope, with the 'e' being the cancer ribbon, would be a permanent reminder, and a bold, positive response to the physical and emotional marks lung cancer has left on my body.

I also started thinking about a second tattoo—the tree of life. I wanted to incorporate my mom, dad and aunt (whom I lost to lung cancer) and Jason, Jack, Shae, Meg and Maya (my husband and kids)—all of whom inspire me to fight every day. Like a family tree showing deep roots and branches that connect to me, with a symbol (a leaf) for each person, this tattoo would symbolize love and eternal life.

My kids are 17, 16, 14 and 11 so I thought about what their response would be (you would never approve of us getting a tattoo…) and the message I would be sending them. When I got the response I suspected, I simply said that they were right; I would not approve of them getting a tattoo. I told them that they are far too young to know what they would want forever or to understand the impact of a permanent decision. I explained that at my age, with my life experiences, I know this is something I want for the rest of my life.

I got my tattoos two weeks ago. I went with some of my cousins and nieces, but my biggest supporter, who was by my side the whole time, was my 16-year-old daughter Shae. I was nervous about the pain, but every time I brought it up Shae would remind me of the worst pain I have ever felt—having the chest tubes removed after my first lung cancer surgery. She also reminded me that lung cancer has caused me a lot more pain over the years and that is the exact reason I was getting the tattoos!

The HOPE tattoo on my inner left wrist is my anchor; it reminds me that hope, faith and the love of my family and friends got me through those darkest moments and will do so again when I need strength and courage. I was going to get this tattoo in a place that could be easily covered, but doing so would have taken away its significance. The tattoo is a statement that I believe in to my core. I want people to ask me about it so I can share my story and raise awareness about lung cancer. And for me personally, every morning when I wake up, throughout the day and every night before I go to bed, I want to see that permanent reminder that there is always Hope!

The tree of life tattoo on my front hip is my rock, my strength. It represents the closest people to my heart, for whom I live for and fight for every day. It reminds me of where I came from, where I have been and how far I have come. It is especially comforting to know that my mom, dad and aunt are always with me.

I am still a little surprised that I actually got 'inked', but I don't regret it one bit. In fact, it's quite the opposite. I love my tattoos. The stories and meanings behind them are connected deeply to my heart, so much so that I actually marked my body with them—something I thought I would never do. Never say never...

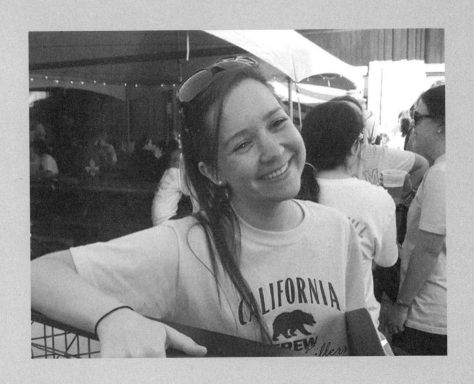

8

Jill Costello

On the occasion of *Sports Illustrated*'s sixtieth anniversary, the magazine selected its sixty greatest articles. One of these, which ran in the November 29, 2010 issue, was entitled "The Courage of Jill Costello."

"It started as a dull ache in Jill Costello's abdomen, the kind you get after a night of suspect Chinese food," the article began. "Only it didn't go away. It was June 2009, and the Cal crew had just returned from the NCAA championships in Cherry Hill, N.J. The Bears had finished second, behind Stanford, continuing a remarkable run of six top four finishes in seven years."

Jill was about to begin something even more remarkable on a road that began with the devastating news that the pain in her abdomen was actually lung cancer that had spread to multiple parts of her body. The odds weren't good, and this story doesn't end with a Hollywood finish, either for the Cal Berkley woman's crew team or Jill herself.

Or maybe it does

"She squeezed a lifetime into her twenty-one years," says her mother, Mary, as Jill's father, Jim, looks on. "She affected, and continues to affect, so many people, putting a face on how lung cancer can strike an otherwise perfectly healthy young woman who never smoked. We took her to the emergency room on Father's Day in June of 2010. She was so sick and she was in a lot of pain. I asked her what she hoped from this hospitalization?"

"'A cure,' Jill told me."

Jim and Mary hadn't been to the annual gala the Addario Lung Cancer Foundation (now the GO2 Foundation, following our merger with the Lung Cancer Alliance) holds every year in San Francisco for a while. But they came in 2019, and we made plans to talk in the last feverish moments of setup, even as the waitstaff finished setting the hundred or so tables in the ballroom. We stake out a quiet sitting area where the cocktail reception will be starting soon.

"She still believed, she still fought," Mary continues, "but two days later she said she was done fighting and wasn't afraid. Jill was in control right to the end."

It was so oddly and ironically appropriate that Jill made her mark on the Cal rowing team in the crucial role of coxswain (pronounced "cox-in"), the person who's in charge of the boat from a seat in the very front facing the rowers. Setting the pace, controlling navigation and steering. The person running the show, just as Jill ran her own life.

"She was determined to succeed in everything she went into," Mary resumes, "and she never turned down a challenge. When Jill had chemotherapy, Jim, my sister Cathy, and I would all spend the whole day in the hospital with her. I can remember one time she brought a tote bag with her."

"'What's that for?' I asked her."

"'I'm going back to Berkeley once we're finished here.'"

"'Is there something really important you need to get back to school for?'"

"'Yes, my life.'"

"Lung cancer," Mary tells me, holding Jim's hand, "was a part of her life, but she never let it define her."

"She treated cancer like something else on her plate," Jim adds. "Something else she needed to deal with."

And that was, through the time of her treatment as well as before, a pretty crowded plate. Indeed, Jill had set three goals for herself, and nothing, including cancer, was going to change them: graduate from Cal Berkeley, serve as coxswain for the varsity boat, and win Nationals. She achieved the first two and came within mere inches of the third as well, the Bears finishing runner-up for the second year in a row.

Mary nods when we come to that. "They'd come so close and all the girls were crying. They wanted to win so badly, for themselves, sure, but especially for Jill. But Jill was smiling, trying to cheer them up. Telling the girls there was nothing more they could have done, just as she had in her fight with cancer. They'd won the Pac-10 championship prior to Nationals, and that smile on Jill's face as she hoisted the trophy overhead…"

How she came to cox Cal's first boat that day is another testament to Jill's grit and determination, how she never let cancer beat her.

"Her first practice back was a Saturday morning in early March at Briones Reservoir, fifteen minutes from the Cal campus," that *Sports Illustrated* article continues. "The team began with a two-mile jog, from the boathouse to the reservoir entrance and back. Jill sat in the boathouse clutching a cup of tea and watched as, one mile out, her teammates began changing color. All fifty of them tore off their sweatshirts to reveal yellow T-shirts that read CAL CREW CANCER KILLERS. All doubts she had about her decision vanished in the cool morning air. After Jill's first practice the girls in her boat went up to [Coach] O'Neill. Jill, they told him, had been awesome. Not because she was courageous or because she had made it through practice. Rather, because she was now a better coxswain. And as the weeks went on, O'Neill realized the rowers were right. He likes to say that there are three types of coxswain: the motivator, always rah-rah; the drill sergeant, ever demanding peak performance; and the airline pilot, cool and collected. Her first three years, Jill was more of a motivator, but now she had become an airline pilot. Maybe it was the cancer, maybe it was maturity, maybe it was a combination of the two. No matter what happened—a missed stroke, a slow start—Jill did not change her tenor. It would all be O.K., she seemed to say."

When O'Neill gave them a say in the matter, teammates voted her into the first boat and never looked back.

Jill came to the Living Room the very night she graduated college. It wasn't enough for her just to beat cancer herself; she wanted to beat cancer period. I remember getting a call from Jill in December of 2009, six months after her diagnosis.

"I want to do a run," she said.

"That's great, Jill!" I said, thinking out loud that the coming summer would be the perfect time.

"It can't wait. We have to do it now."

That was Jill the drill sergeant, in other words. And, needless to say, the run happened and ended up serving as the template for "Jogs for Jill," fundraisers that continue all over the country to this day in her memory and in pursuit of her most passionate cause. That's Jill still being Jill, in this case the rah-rah motivator.

Which brings a reflective smile to Mary's face. "Every time Jill was in the hospital overnight, I stayed with her. I didn't want her to be alone. The first morning, when I woke up, she was watching something on her iPad. She smiled at me and said, 'Come here, get into bed with me. We'll watch this together.' At first, I thought, *How sweet that is. She really needs me.* Then I realized she was comforting me, because she knew I was the one who needed it."

Jill, the airline pilot.

"I remember when Jill was maybe five years old. She was dancing and singing, really putting on a show and showing no signs it was going to end. So I told her, 'Jill, the show is over.' She stared at me and said, 'No, it's not!' For Jill, nothing was over until she said it was." Mary smiles, her gaze a bit distant for a moment. "Everyone wants to believe their child is special. Jim and I are no different there. But I'll tell you a story that typifies Jill's approach to life and to cancer that had become such a big part of it in that last year. For her radiation, a mold of her body was prepared for her to lie in to make sure she didn't move during treatments. When she finished her final treatment, she told the staff she wanted to take the mold with her. I said, 'Jill, why do you want that? I don't want to see or even think about it.' But she insisted that we put the mold in the car and take it with us in the drive back to Berkeley. We parked in front of the sorority and her sisters went and got this stick with all these ribbons hanging from it. Then they turned the radiation mold into a piñata and just bashed the heck out of it, like she was going to do with cancer. 'I'm going to take this and beat it to shit.' That was her attitude until those last two days, and that's what her sorority sisters did to that body mold."

That fall, Jill had been selected to chair the entire sorority rush process at Cal Berkeley, no easy task on a campus dominated by the Greek system. As with everything else, Jill attacked the role with her customary passion and drive. Adding more to her plate, what with classes and training, seemed to make her stronger, not weaker.

K. C. Oakley, Jill's sorority sister, best friend, and a fellow standout athlete, wasn't surprised. K. C. couldn't be with us at the gala, but I caught up with her later to get her thoughts on what made Jill so special.

"I was in the hospital the day she was diagnosed," K. C. recalls. "She pulled us into the room right afterwards and said, 'I've been diagnosed with lung cancer, and I don't want you guys to look at the statistics.' She knew immediately how we'd react if we heard what she'd just heard about her chances, and she didn't want the focus to be on that. She took this as another time to fight instead of worry about numbers. What she was doing was creating this militia around her that wasn't going to get run down or beaten by the disease. Jill's ultimate goal would have been to still be alive today, still fighting lung cancer, not just for herself, but for everyone."

A champion skier with Olympic aspirations, K. C. won the 2011 North American Grand Prix Cup as well as the Silver Medal at the 2011 US National Championships. That same year she qualified for the World Cup Finals and finished ninth overall in the World Cup rankings, feats that placed her on firm footing to make a run at the 2014 Winter Olympic Games in Sochi, Russia. But exacerbating struggles against a nerve injury in her lower legs and a condition called exertional compartment syndrome forced her into surgery and ended her Olympic dreams, for 2014 anyway. I ask her if Jill's memory helped her deal with her own disappointments and setbacks.

"Sure, in the sense that I knew that no matter how bad things seemed, it could have been a lot worse. Thinking about Jill always made—*makes*—the highs higher and the lows seem not as low. Would I have given up the Olympics, given up everything, to get Jill back? Absolutely. It comes down to perspective. You lose a person you talk to every day, it becomes this hole you can't fill. Not going to the Olympics didn't create a hole; it was just something to maneuver around. I can remember whenever Jill was in the hospital, the corridor would be lined with friends and sorority sisters sitting on the floor playing cards while waiting for their chance to see her. We could only let a few in at a time and make sure they didn't stay too long, because we had to keep in mind how sick she was."

K. C. went on to get her MBA and is now working at Goldman Sachs, where she "integrates holistic life techniques into comprehensive financial, tax and estate, and philanthropic planning for a small number of entrepreneurs, wealthy families, and foundations so they not only match their needs but also lifestyles and lifetime goals."

Did such a unique approach to wealth management derive from her relationship with Jill?

"I didn't go train the summer Jill got diagnosed. I just couldn't be away from her. You have to do what's right and best for you at the time. My goals, my priorities, needed to be changed. Everything changes when you become a caregiver, and skiing was nothing for me compared to my best friend. I think that taught me about the importance of balance. There's a lot of bad happening, but a lot of good can come out of it, and being adaptable is so important. You need to look at the finer details of how someone lives, the avenues they need to explore because of the kind of person they are."

K. C. is also a founding member of Jill's Legacy, which has as its motto, BEAT LUNG CANCER BIG TIME! The Jogs for Jill runs Jill started herself have become a nationwide fundraising phenomenon, but that wouldn't be enough for Jill, as K. C. quickly points out.

"She wanted to take Jogs for Jill international. She had this quality of bossiness, but it was bossy because she knew what she wanted to get out of any situation. And she never said no to anything, always looking for new opportunities and was down for any adventure. She wasn't good at everything she did—don't get me started on her singing and dancing!—but she always tried. She was a doer, and she wanted to beat cancer, not just for herself, but for everyone. I'm getting married in a month, and my bridesmaids were the people who were there by her side right until the end. They weren't my best friends when Jill was diagnosed, but they became my best friends because of who they proved themselves to be."

Mary knows that was the effect Jill had on people, leading by example.

"There's this huge mountain in Yosemite National Park called Half Dome, and it's a big thing to climb it. The crew team went there every year to climb to the top of Half Dome to build camaraderie. And for the first three years on the team, Jill had climbed Half Dome."

"Ran up it," Jim swiftly corrects.

"When you're on top you can see things you can't see from anywhere else, any other vantage point, just like Jill's cancer gave her a whole new perspective on life. 'I'm not afraid,' she'd always say, even though there was nothing more she could or that anybody could do. That final race, when Cal came in second in the Nationals, she knew they were winners because they'd done everything they could possibly do and just came up a little short in the end. Just like Jill did in her fight against cancer."

One of her last wishes was to create a lasting memory at St. Ignatius Prep, the high school she attended in San Francisco, in the form of a tree that could weather any storm life threw at it and stay strong. But the school prided itself on its already plentiful landscaping and was concerned about the precedent that might set, so they politely declined.

"Then," Mary says, picking up the story there, "we had this terrible storm and the wind uprooted one of their trees. The next week the school called me and asked if the offer to donate a tree in Jill's name was still on the table."

"See," K. C. Oakley smiles, when I tell her that story, "Jill always gets her way."

Mary and Jim both smile at that notion too.

"It would be a great consolation to Jill that her life led to helping other people," Mary says. "When she realized right at the end that she wasn't going to survive, she wrote in her journal, 'Did I make the world a better place? Yes, I did.' I think she always demanded the best of herself, challenged herself to be the best she could be. And because she was that way, she made the people around her want to be their best too. Anything else would have been disappointing to her, and second best didn't exist in her vocabulary."

To the point where shortly before what was to be Jill's final race, the family made a pilgrimage to Lourdes in France, site of numerous purported miracles over the ages.

"It was an incredible experience," Mary recalls. "We went with the Knights of Malta, who sponsor sick people, twenty-five thousand from all over the world they refer to as *Malades*. But the odds of getting to Lourdes were long at best. It's a huge process to be selected. You have to write letters, find sponsors from the religious and medical community. It's almost impossible, yet when the selection committee read Jill's letter it was unanimous. We went to Lourdes and would have loved to have come home with a physical miracle, and in a way I suppose we did. No, we didn't return with a physical cure; we came home with a feeling of peace. A strange feeling that left us believing that so many people are facing devastating challenges and they all have faith, looking for a miracle in whatever form that takes. We came home secure in the notion we were doing everything we could physically. Seeking out every doctor, every treatment, anything to keep Jill healthy. Sometimes, though, we have to realize it's out of our hands and in God's. It wasn't for us to determine Jill's fate."

In addition to that inner peace, Jill and her family came back with something else from Lourdes: a supply of the famed holy water that Jill swiftly dispensed to her teammates on the eve of the Nationals. If Lourdes couldn't deliver her wish to live, perhaps it could help deliver another one: for her beloved Bears to be crowned national champions.

It wasn't desperation that sent the Costellos to Lourdes, it was hope. Jill never lost hope until the very, very end, and that more than anything was responsible for her squeezing ten years of living into those final twelve months. You think about stage IV lung cancer patients and maybe the first thing that comes to mind is how desperate they must be. Not in my experience. Hope and faith really were the best medicine for Jill and far too many like her. The difference is that more progress has been made therapeutically since Jill lost her battle in June of 2010 than in the forty years previous when President Nixon declared war on cancer in 1971. And if comparable progress continues to be made over the next decade, lung cancer patients won't have to go to Lourdes in search of a miracle because there will be one waiting for them at the hospital around the corner. And if you're reading this and you're sick, you should know you don't have to go it alone, just like Jill didn't go it alone. The lung cancer community is immensely supportive, one great big family drawn together by a common experience none of us wanted to have. We're a giant support group and we are there for you, just like Jill would have been.

Jill spoke at Genentech, the cancer research firm that continues to develop drugs aimed at making lung cancer a manageable disease. She was interviewed on NPR as the voice of nonsmoking lung cancer sufferers. She became the national face of eradicating the stigma that only smokers contract the disease.

"I think she felt you put one foot in front of the other," Mary says.

"Life is happening now," Jim adds. "That encapsulates everything a cancer patient needs to know."

"Do what you have to. Not tomorrow or a week from now, but today."

Mary should know. Since Jill's passing, she's been treated twice for cancer, first uterine and then breast, in 2016.

"Just thinking of her, knowing she was there with me, helped me so much when I was going through chemo and radiation, reminding me that cancer wasn't my life, just a part of my life. I never felt overwhelmed. That helped me immensely as an adult suffering from cancer, never mind a younger person. I was going to enjoy the future in a way Jill never got to experience."

As was the case for her daughter, cancer only rented space in her body; it never took ownership any more than it did for Jill right up until the end. Call that Jill the motivator again, or perhaps Jill the airline pilot, maybe even Jill the drill sergeant.

"In June of 2010, Jill was graduating college and, I have to say, that after a year of cancer, all the chemo and everything that goes with that, all the emotions, I wasn't in a party mood. But Jill wanted to have a party, and I have to think my daughter has taught me so much because she taught me that you need to celebrate, you always need to celebrate, whether there's cancer in the picture or not."

And, I know this won't surprise you, she had a plan for the future.

"Jill was part of something larger than herself now," that brilliant *Sports Illustrated* article continues. "For six months she'd been working with the San Francisco-based Bonnie J. Addario Lung Cancer Foundation, and she had agreed to become its director of public awareness after graduation. She funneled her energy into organizing a charity run in Golden Gate Park called Jog for Jill, which when it was held on a foggy Sunday in September of 2010 would attract close to 5,000 people and raise more than $320,000. She continued her schoolwork at Cal, as diligent as ever. When, after a therapy-related extension, she handed in her final paper in International Trade, her professor gave her an A-minus without even looking at Jill's work. Naturally Jill was upset, believing she'd turned in a really good paper, one she'd worked hard on to finish. She contacted the professor, who took a look and awarded her a straight A. The result: Jill had a 4.0 average in her final semester at Cal."

One of the last times I saw Jill, I noticed a telltale bulge in her abdomen, indicative of a swollen liver that's normally a clear sign the end is near. Right alongside her sat the Maltese puppy I'd given her as a graduation present. She named the dog Jack. Get it? Jack and Jill. She was buoyant and hopeful to the end.

I ask Jim and Mary to give me their three wishes for the future.

"I wish there'd be a cure for all cancers," Mary chimes in immediately. "And I wish people would recognize other people's pain and be kind."

"I wish lung cancer didn't have the stigma that goes with it," Jim interjects. "Anybody can get it at any time. That lesson is Jill's greatest legacy."

Mary nods. "We still go every year when Cal takes on Stanford in the penultimate race of the season. People, total strangers, come up to us and they all know Jill's story and it's influenced them so much beyond cancer. Everyone's going to have some challenge in their life, cancer or something else. Don't let that challenge consume you and become your life. Face it and go on with what's really important to you."

"That first race we went to after Jill passed," she reflects softly, after a pause, "both teams whipped off their warm-up tops to reveal matching T-shirts that read BEAT LUNG CANCER. How much Jill would have loved that because that's what her goal was. Maybe not for herself, but for somebody else."

I'm alive today in large part thanks to Dr. Melissa Lim. It was Melissa, a lung cancer specialist at Redwood Pulmonary Medical Associates, who referred me to Dr. David Jablons, the surgeon who saved my life on the operating table. When we spoke, I asked Melissa five questions pertaining to the state of lung cancer treatment today.

1. Based on where we are today compared to five or ten years ago, where do you think we'll be or where might we be in ten years?

Treatment is definitely going to be more individualized, and I expect us to get better at the diagnostic part. The challenge we face, and what has always struck me about lung cancer, is how heterogenous the disease is. It's actually a collection of different diseases, and I think we're going to get better at identifying what makes the disease different and how we individualize treatments to provide patients with a more positive prognosis and outcomes. Too often the statistics associated with lung cancer give patients a more fatalistic view of those outcomes. But by educating both providers and patients on the true state of care and the importance of individualized treatment, we can give people realistic hope.

2. What's the first thing you say to a just or recently diagnosed lung cancer patient?

Whenever you use the word "cancer," people don't hear anything you say after that. So it's really important not to talk over people. Just start by giving them space after you've given them the initial diagnosis. But I also tell them that no matter what that diagnosis is, it will be treatable. I think it's really important that we give people that hope and we don't become nihilistic about population statistics. It's important to let them know they have options and that there are lung cancer survivors they can talk to about this, and that it's their specific DNA fingerprints that will ultimately determine what treatment choice may be available to them.

3. What surprises/impresses you most about the lung cancer patients you treat?

It surprises me that such a wide variety of people are affected by this disease. The number of people who have lung cancer who never smoked is growing, so an already common disease is becoming even more common. And it's surprising to us as providers how lung cancer can behave so unpredictably. There's so much we've yet to learn because of that heterogenous nature of the disease—why it's behaving so aggressively in one person, yet so indolently in another.

4. Are we headed for a time when lung cancer screening becomes more common and effective?

A recent study of an extremely targeted group of smokers and former smokers between the ages of fifty-five and eighty showed a 20 percent reduction in mortality in the targeted group. A tougher issue to face when it comes to screening is how best to identify known risk factors. But if you apply screening too broadly, more people will die of complications from the screening than the cancer itself. Screening comes with risks of its own. So we need to develop better blood screening tools instead of relying on radiographic tools. We need to find tumors earlier in their development, as opposed to later.

5. What's your biggest hope for the future?

What we're hoping is that the next wave of treatments for lung cancer and cancer in general will be able to morph the disease into something more like HIV, so we can keep it at bay longer and longer. And more and more treatments are coming out toward that end. Looking at this another way, my biggest wish for the future is to be treating fewer people because the disease won't be as prevalent and the patients I do see will be diagnosed at an earlier stage.

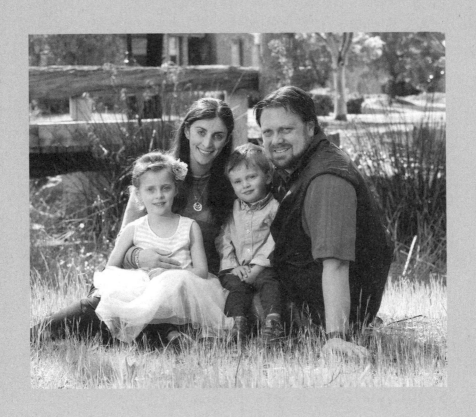

9

Lisa Briggs

"My husband and I took our kids to Disney World not too long ago," Lisa Briggs tells me, "and more than anything else, lung cancer reminds me of being on a roller coaster that's whipping you around at high speeds, a hundred feet up in the air."

Considering that Lisa was diagnosed just four months after giving birth to her son and had been suffering worsening symptoms of the disease throughout her pregnancy, maybe closer to a thousand feet and spinning at centrifugal-force speeds would be a more accurate way of putting it.

"When I was first diagnosed, it was a very critical situation because there was a significant amount of bleeding in my lungs. And if my doctors couldn't stop that bleeding, I was going to die. I felt like I had not only gotten on the wrong ride but that it was now about to crash, and I was completely shaken and confused."

Like many lung cancer sufferers, she was misdiagnosed for a considerable amount of time. In Lisa's case, doctors initially attributed her symptoms to the added pressure of her abdomen on the lungs and rib cage due to her pregnancy. That is, until she coughed up blood in front of her toddler daughter and infant son.

"My GP sent me straight to hospital where some tests were performed," she wrote for Lung Foundation Australia in October 2017, "which initially indicated bronchitis, but when I continued to cough up blood for three days continuously, my doctor recommended further tests, which finally confirmed the real reason for my symptoms—a tumor in my right lung which was wrapped around and strangling one of my heart's main arteries. By this stage, I needed emergency surgery to stop the bleeding in my lungs, and I was told there was no guarantee this would be successful. Thankfully, it was. While I was lucky to have survived, further tests and examination in hospital soon after revealed the lung cancer had already spread to eight different locations in my body, and it was then that I was told there was no cure. Initially I felt numb and then the emotions began to snowball. The panic set in, followed by feelings of helplessness, fear, and confusion all rolled into one. My life as I once knew it was totally falling apart and the fear of losing my life was devastating. I was scared for my husband Kirk and my children."

I remind her of that blog she wrote for Lung Foundation Australia, quoting from it, and she picks the story up from there over our Skype call. "My daughter was at a critical age of development, while my four-month-old son was so heavily dependent on me at the time—he was exclusively breastfed—and all of that suddenly came to a complete stop. Their security blanket was completely ripped away! The thoughts of my children growing up without their mum or without memories of me was paralyzing. Then to think that my husband might not wake in the mornings with me by his side, or the thoughts of him having to take on the role of being both the mum and the dad, was heartbreaking.

"But here I was hospitalized, with nurses coming in several times a day while I pump out my milk and discard it. Back home, my son wasn't eating because he was used to the breast, not the bottle, and I was in the hospital too sick to do anything practical about it. After I was rushed in, I was told to stop taking all my medications, which included a contraceptive pill. But only a few weeks later, it was in fact this advice which precluded me from being a participant of a clinical trial, which I would have otherwise been eligible for, because I needed to be on the pill for three consecutive months. No one had thought that far ahead. Thankfully, we found an alternative solution to this issue, but there were a lot of setbacks initially."

But Lisa Briggs overcame those and more. One of my favorite quotes comes from Nelson Mandela: "It seems impossible until it is done." Some lung cancer sufferers seem comfortable cast in the role of victim, while others choose not to be defined by the disease so much as the courage it takes to move forward. And no one exemplifies that better than Lisa, whom I recently Skyped with all the way from Australia.

"Continuing the roller-coaster metaphor," she says, "my lung cancer came with so many highs and lows, dips and darts, with no warning of when the next sharp drop or rise was going to come. It's not just riding a roller coaster, it's riding a roller coaster with your eyes closed and no foresight for what's coming next. Now that I'm living a reasonably normal life, I prefer to focus on the highs: the clinical trial I was ultimately able to get into and the time that drug has given me I otherwise never would have had to see my children reach milestones and spend quality time with them and my husband. The dreams that I have can come true now, and without the cutting-edge therapy I received, I wouldn't be here talking to you. I've connected with some of the most amazing oncologists who were full of compassion and surrounded by people who sacrifice their own time to help patients. Another high—and I owe this to you, Bonnie—is using my own story to give other people hope. But there's no greater high than when the treatment actually works. Labored breathing becomes normal again, life itself becomes normal again, and suddenly my children and my husband have their mum and wife back in their lives again.

"Then there are the lows, starting with the initial diagnosis that makes you feel like you're facing a death sentence. Navigating the health care system in Australia was horrendous; like riding a roller coaster for the very first time, to continue with that metaphor, you know a big drop is coming, but you don't know when. Anxiety caused by the unexpected becomes a constant. You don't have someone there to support you, hold your hand, and tell you everything's going to be okay, because nobody's really sure. And it goes even deeper than that, to the practical side of things. I was looked after by a multidisciplinary team of surgeons, oncologists, and radiologists, and I was bombarded by visits from the person in charge of each team accompanied into my room by a group of subordinates. It seemed as soon as one group left, another entered—nonstop. Meanwhile, as good as these doctors were individually, there was no single entity collating all that information and taking charge, which has practical consequences on top of the emotional ones."

Lisa's voice cracks here. I get the sense that in retelling the story, she's also reliving it, riddled by all that stress and uncertainty again. She speaks with amazing eloquence and uses vivid imagery to help tell her story, almost like she's a character in someone else's book trying to figure out how to escape the pages.

"Once," Lisa continues, "I was told I was going to have a PET scan to see if my cancer had spread, as this was crucial to my treatment plan. But the day of my scan the imaging department had no record that I'd be coming in. No one had told them, and to make matters worse, the machine was closed for maintenance that day—at least until my very passionate Italian family convinced the nuclear medicine department to restart the machine once maintenance was complete so I could have my scan as scheduled. The other really frustrating things were the delays in treatment at Christmastime. I'd been told I wouldn't be able to start the clinical trial I'd been approved for until January fifth. Two or three extra weeks is a lifetime when you're fighting cancer, and every minute counts, never mind every day. I'd coughed up blood two more times recently and really began to think that I was going to die."

She stops to compose herself. I can hear Lisa breathing quietly on the other end of the Skype line. I picture her vital, effervescent personality and think this is what it took to throttle her, something as big and bad as lung cancer. Then she clears her throat and resumes.

"I went into my daughter's room. 'Jasmine,' I said, shaking her, 'wake up, wake up. Mommy needs to talk to you.'"

The little girl stirred, then whined and pushed her away.

"'Please wake up. Mommy needs to talk to you and it's really important.'"

"Finally, she opened her eyes all the way, regarding me in all that childhood innocence. 'What's wrong, Mum?' she asked, having seen the despair in my eyes."

"'Mommy loves you with all her heart. No matter what happens, I want you to always remember how much I love you.'"

"I was basically saying goodbye to my daughter because I didn't think I was going to make it long enough to start that clinical trial."

But she did; the roller coaster that had become her life leveled out just in time.

"It wasn't my time to go," Lisa adds.

"Do you remember how we met?" I ask her, figuring it's a good time to change the subject.

"You bet. Among all the things I experienced on the roller coaster was that once you're outside the hospital system, there was very little support out there for patients living with lung cancer. I could find only two face-to-face support groups—*two*, in the entire country—and they were located in other Australian states, too far for me to travel in my condition. That's in contrast to hundreds for prostate and breast cancer."

Stunned by those numbers, I ask Lisa to repeat them.

"It took me twelve months before I finally came to Lung Foundation Australia. You'll remember that I was interviewed for a newspaper article that led the foundation to contact me, and in that discussion the reporter mentioned the ALK and ROS1 in Australia Facebook group. And it was a member of that group who told me to contact you as someone I had to talk to because you were a leader in the field. She told me I had to reach out to you, that you were doing a genomic study on young lung cancer patients and I fit all the criteria of the subjects they were looking for. I was overwhelmed, didn't know where to go or what to do, like when you have a crush on a boy and don't know how to approach him for fear of saying the wrong thing. I finally reached out and sent you an email. Well, oh my gosh, I was gobsmacked by your response. You talked to me for over an hour and sent me all the paperwork I needed to be part of your study. You sent me vials for blood collection, remember?"

"I remember they were rejected by Australian Customs, so you never got them. But I told you not to worry."

"Right. Because I wanted to come to America anyway and this gave me an excuse. I'd lost a friend who had a child my son's age. My husband and I decided to take a family trip to Disney World, and I wasn't going to put it off any longer. We came to San Francisco from Florida, and you sent a phlebotomist to my hotel room and he drew my blood for your study right there. Later that morning you sent a car to pick me up so we could actually meet each other."

When that happened, we hugged so long I thought we'd never let go. Two strangers who'd never seen each other before locked in an embrace neither of us wanted to break. As if we were both on that roller coaster now and needed to cling to one another to avoid falling off in the middle of the ride.

"I've never felt anything like that," Lisa adds. "The hope, the love, the support. The unspoken compassion and empathy were like nothing I'd ever experienced before. We chatted for hours. 'Hey,' you said at one point, 'let's do a Facebook Live event.' And that's what we did, right then and there in your Living Room. My husband and children joined in too. It was really powerful and got great comments from the viewers.

Then we went out for lunch. If I've never told you this before, you've been a second mum to me ever since."

Two years later, my foundation was coordinating a fundraising walk we call Your Next Step Is the Cure. Lisa and her family had decided to return to the US and insisted on participating. She extended her family's stay in the US, just so she could join in, but then severe rainstorms shut the whole thing down. Nevertheless, we still raised a lot of money, and it gave us an excuse to spend more time together, just Lisa and me.

There's definitely an intrinsic bond between and among lung cancer survivors. We're members, after all, of a very exclusive club. Given the much higher lung cancer mortality rates not all that long ago, in the past there really wasn't even a club whose members have shared an experience no one else can really relate to. Lisa's considerably younger than I and, obviously, was diagnosed much younger than I was. While my own kids are just about her age, I can relate so well to her because our children were first and foremost on our minds when we began treatment, regardless of age, providing both motivation and inspiration. Plenty of lung cancer patients have adult children, and our tendency is to not want to burden them, just as younger patients with younger children count maintaining a degree of household normalcy a high priority. It's yet another dynamic that many of us have no choice but to face as we and our families adjust to the new normal.

That said, the new normal forced upon Lisa by her lung cancer treatment presented an entirely different set of challenges.

"My daughter had always been a bright, energetic little girl. But after I got sick, she went into a shell, only wanted to play by herself. No three-year-old should have to go through that, to be there when her mum coughs up blood. My son was only four months old, and he'd go to child care every day to provide normalcy and routine for his life, but he didn't see me enough to even know who his mum was. When he was eight months old or so, I'd drop him off and he'd practically jump out of my arms to go to the child care workers. They were the ones giving him nurturing at the time, not me. It's hard to see that your son would rather be in someone else's arms than your own. My daughter said 'Mama' at nine months. But my son was fifteen months old and still hadn't. We'd gone camping that weekend, and all of a sudden I heard him say 'Mama!' in the back of the caravan."

"'Are you going to go to him?' my husband asked."

"'No,'" I told him. "'I'm going to sit here with a huge smile on my face and listen to him call it over and over again.'"

"It was one of the best moments in my life. Having not had him in my care full time, the way I had to parent him was different. He didn't always know how to respond to me, and I didn't know how to respond to him. At times, it felt more like I'd adopted a child instead of nurtured my own."

One of the unspoken costs of cancer, which tends to rewrite the rules of everything we'd taken for granted prior to getting sick, is you have to find a new way to be a parent, be a family. There's no sugar-coating that pill, except to say the good news is that more and more patients are living long enough to confront these new challenges that never existed when people died before they had to adjust to the new normal. I know that they would have given anything to live and enjoy making that adjustment.

Lisa's daughter is about to turn eight and her son is now four and a half. As we speak, she emails me a recent class project of his, entitled ALL ABOUT MY MUM, with the blanks filled in:

Mum's favorite thing to do is…snuggle with us.

Her favorite food is…pizza.

We like to…play toys…*together.*

Mum is really good at…doing yoga.

Mum is not very good at…getting ink for the computer.

Mum always says…she loves me, Jas, and Dad.

The best thing about my Mum is…I like drawing with her and playing Lego.

"I don't know what the teacher thought, but I know that if pre-schoolers got grades, he'd get an A+ from his mum!"

There's a video on YouTube of Lisa called "Just One Breath" in which early on she says, "The sun is up and it's a new day." I ask her what that means.

"It's actually about more than that now. It's about the sun, flowers, and rainbows, particularly the rainbow of hope. When I first got sick, I was happy just to see the sun come up. Now, I want to see more. I want to see the rainbow."

By her own description, until the lung cancer she was always known as a bubbly, effervescent personality. I ask her if the whole experience had changed that.

"No, not at all. It's made me appreciate life more, while not taking away who I am. My identity is still the same. Sure, there are times when I feel more fatigued than others, but that will never take the smile from my face because I've got too much to live for. Who I am will never change. I just view myself, and life, through a different lens now. I'm especially partial to the image of the rainbow because I often talk about the fact that lung cancer is somewhat doom and gloom, like it's always raining and the sun never comes out, overshadowed by the dark clouds that loom above. But when you look deeper, patients are actually like raindrops, and all the research and treatment make up the sun shining down from above. And when the sun shines through those dark clouds, onto the delicate raindrops, we get our rainbow of hope, which represents where I am in my life right now."

Lisa's Facebook page is called "CONQUERING CANCER: Develop YOUR Will to LIVE." Her hashtag is @LivingLife82. Her posts, while not voluminous, are always pointed and heartfelt, normally directed at fellow lung cancer patients and cheering the new therapies that are keeping them alive.

In that video I mentioned earlier, a healthy Lisa Briggs is pictured pushing her son and daughter on matching swings, going back and forth between them. As I watch it, it strikes me that no matter how hard she pushes, her children never loop over the top, remaining safe and secure.

Lisa sees it a different way.

"I want my children to experience as many highs with me as possible because I'm keenly aware I might not always be with them. You just never know. We try and condense what we have into a small package of time crammed with those experiences we desperately want to do. No matter how hard I push, I can't make that happen any quicker or better. No matter how high I push those swings, they're never going to come all the way around. And no matter how much you try to condense those moments, it's not always going to result in the best outcome down the road. It's more important to sit back and just keep pushing the swing."

My daughter Danielle serves as chief patient officer now for the GO2 Foundation for Lung Cancer. She oversees all patient support and services, including the one-on-ones we arrange for lung cancer patients, all the education programs, and the Living Room broadcasts themselves. Her article below offers a heartfelt look into the vast number of those whose lives have been affected and changed by the disease without suffering from it themselves. Because when a family member gets cancer, the whole family gets cancer.

A CAREGIVER'S VIEW

I became a caregiver when my mom was diagnosed with stage IIIB lung cancer in 2004. It was one of the most terrifying things I had ever had to face until that point in my life. She was only in her fifties. I had three small children, and I couldn't fathom her not being a part of their lives. One of the hardest things about this for me was not the chemo or radiation or even seeing her so sick—it was the fear I had of losing her. The fear of no longer having Sunday dinners or family vacations. The fear that my youngest son, who was only three at the time, would not remember her. The fear that the matriarch of our family might not beat this disease.

The easy part? The easy part was being able to try, in some small way, to give back all of the love and support she had shown me my entire life. Through good times and bad, she was always there for me. I only thought about being there for her, however I could. She was my rock, and it was my turn to try and be hers.

For the most part, Mom was an easy patient. She was strong and quite often hid how she was actually feeling with forced laughter and a smile—especially when the grandkids were around. Forever the fighter, forever the warrior. Some days, though, were harder than others. Like the day she, my sister, and I shaved her head, or the long days in the infusion rooms watching the chemo drip for hours. The radiation burns and all of the other side effects. The days she simply didn't want to get out of bed and would beg us to leave her alone. The days when she looked so weak, so fragile, and so scared…those days were hard.

We tried to support our mom in any way we could. We mostly listened to her. Her wants and needs changed throughout the process, and we in turn changed accordingly. When she didn't feel like eating (refused actually), we would keep trying different things until finally she would relent and take a few bites. When she didn't want to get out of bed, we would coax her out with a promise that if she'd just take a few steps, we would leave her be. When she didn't feel like smiling, we'd bring in one of her grandchildren (or all nine) as a reminder that there was always a reason to smile.

The funny thing about being a caregiver, in whatever way I may have been, is that what she gave me during that time was more meaningful than anything I could have done for her. Without even knowing it, she was the one who gave me the strength I needed to be there for her. Actually, she gave me that strength long before she got cancer. She taught me how to be strong, how not to ever give up, and how to persevere even in the toughest of times. She taught me how to love. In a strange way, we were taking care of each other, and although I wish she never got cancer, it was a beautiful thing.

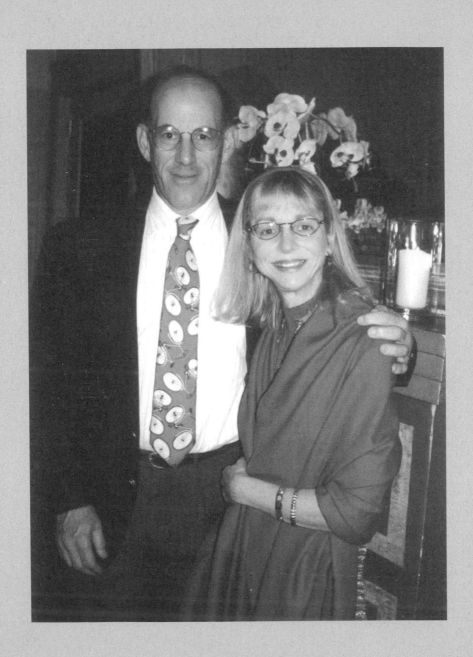

10

Evy and Neil Schiffman

Whenever Neil Schiffman biked, and that included across the entire United States on top of running two Boston Marathons and completing three Ironman competitions, "I set the pace," he said in a 2015 video made by the pharmaceutical giant Eli Lilly during his treatment for stage IV lung cancer. "I've been living for three and a half years with this disease and I still set the pace; it might not be quite as fast, but that's okay. I've come to look at every day as bonus time. My wife, Evy, is my first caretaker and our dog, Cubby, is my second. I can't do all the activities I used to do, so I do other things, like hiking instead of biking. Having cancer isn't going to stop me from being competitive."

And he was quick to point out that he always beat his friends to the top of the mountain.

"He's a role model for how you take on a tough problem," Evy said in the same video. "His attitude is exceptional. He believes this is a doable problem. Playing to win and being positive are his default settings, but cancer is a tough competitor; he just doesn't know if he's going to win yet."

Ultimately, Neil didn't, succumbing to the disease in July 2015. But that's not why Evy is the subject of this chapter. I wanted to highlight her story because not long after she lost Neil, incredibly, she was diagnosed with lung cancer.

She lives on the West Coast too, so we meet in San Carlos, halfway between our homes, for lunch. Our table's not ready, so we begin our talk on a bench outside on a day best described as perfect. As is her custom, Evy doesn't really want to talk about herself right away; she wants to talk about Neil, no longer present physically but still a vital part of her life.

"His entire life—being positive and taking on challenges—that's who Neil was," she reflects with a smile. "And he was that way right up until the last breath he took. I remember an interviewer asking him if, looking back on his life, there was anything he regretted, would have done differently. Neil's answer was that he wished he had better used his capabilities to help other people. He didn't feel he had done enough. So right up until the end he served as a patient advocate. 'We're not just blood,' he'd say, 'we're people. We're not just a smear on a slide, we're people.' He spoke to recently diagnosed lung cancer patients at least twice a week, and that contribution was ever so meaningful to him. He thought the more people he could help in their situation, the more sense he'd be able to make of his own. Neil always felt it's not how fast you do something but how good a person you are, how you reach out to others."

Evy can talk about Neil forever, justifiably so given the kind of person he was. But I want to know how she's doing, so I stop and ask her.

"We were together for forty-three years and complemented each other perfectly. Neil could talk to total strangers for hours on end, and when the conversation ended, they felt like they had learned a lot, that they had connected with him. He was a fountain of knowledge, had an incredible memory, and was brilliant at explaining complicated topics,

like cancer, with clarity and insight. I often thought of him as a transla-
tor, able to synthesize information to the layperson so they really 'got
it.' That's why so many other patients reached out to him to talk.

"What has always been important to me is what David Brooks has
called the Second Mountain: the place where you build close connections, meaningful relationships with other people. I was a high school
English teacher and spent sixteen years in the classroom, and then I
was the communications director for an arts education nonprofit for
twenty-one years. To this day, I am still in touch with some of my
former students, and many of my closest friends are former colleagues.
Now what gets me out of bed in the morning is the volunteer work
I do for your foundation, especially writing those grants that are so
important. That makes me feel like I'm giving something back. Neil
was always there for me, and that loss is irreplaceable. But I also know
that the Addario Foundation [now the GO2 Foundation], and the
caring people who have come into my life because of lung cancer, will
always be there for me."

I remember the first time I met Neil and Evy. It was in the Living
Room. Neil was a leader immediately and patients were drawn to him
from the start. I know that Evy was still in shock about his diagnosis.
She was quiet, happy to sit back and watch Neil interact, and interact
he did. When it was his turn during the Around the Room segment
of the evening, we knew we had someone who was going to be very
involved, not only with us but with the entire community. Evy came
in slowly, in her own way, but she also became a "go-to" person with
her involvement, engaging a bit differently but becoming an equally
big part of our team. I have never met a survivor like Neil since. If he'd
had more time, he would have been on many advisory boards and left
behind an even greater footprint. I miss Neil to this day and consider
both he and Evy to be *familia*.

When I ask Evy about her memories of those early days, her recol-
lections are quite different. "The very first time Neil and I saw you
was from afar; we didn't actually meet you personally," she says. "It

was 2011. We were at your foundation's Your Next Step Is the Cure 5K event in Golden Gate Park. Neil was recently diagnosed and not able to participate, but we wanted to be there, see the event, and learn more about your organization. We heard you speak from the stage and were inspired. We felt the energy and enthusiasm of the participants, patients, and survivors who were there to share hope with each other. I remember saying to Neil that next year, when he felt better, we would put together a team and raise funds for the foundation. He agreed." Evy pauses. "I also remember wondering to myself what our situation would be in a year and if he would even make it. It was so very early in 'our journey' that part of me was still so hesitant about thinking too far into the future. I knew that we would want to participate in 2012, but in my heart I wondered if we would be doing it together or if I would be doing it without him." Evy pauses again. "We were fortunate to participate together, side by side, for the next three years."

So we already knew each other when Evy was diagnosed. With Neil gone, she didn't have any family in the area, so the two of us talked a lot and when she needed someone to go with her to the doctor, to provide a second voice and compassionate ear, one of my daughters, Danielle or Andrea, went with her.

She nods as we talk about that. "The hardest thing for me about having lung cancer wasn't the lung cancer, it was not having Neil here with me. He saw things very clearly about himself and the world, something I always struggle with. The way he thought was sometimes an enigma to me because I overthink everything and I don't have a lot of confidence. Neil always said, 'If your self-worth depends on what someone else tells you, you're never going to be happy.' But I could be me because I had him. It's impossible to realize and truly understand how much someone does for and means to you until they're not there anymore. So many times something will come into my brain and I want to check myself. But there's no one to ask, no one to talk with during dinner."

Evy very likely owes her life to reading a commentary ("Heart screening scan should be available to all," by Dr. David Maron, Dr. William Bommer, and Stephen Shortell, PhD) in her local newspaper. The commentary made the case for universal insurance coverage of a coronary artery calcium CT scan to detect heart attack and stroke risks. The authors argued that pilots, astronauts, and senior military officers receive the scan to determine fitness for duty; it is also part of the president's annual physical. So Evy requested the test as part of her annual physical with her primary care physician. The CT scan brought good news: she was at low risk for heart attack or stroke. The test also revealed unexpected bad news: a mass in the lower left lobe of her lung.

"I was flabbergasted," Evy recalls. "It didn't even cross my mind for one second that I had lung cancer, especially since I'd just lost Neil. I mean, what are the odds?"

Because the mass was determined to be early stage (IA) lung cancer, this inadvertent finding saved her life. Just a few months after she'd read what turned out to be the lifesaving commentary, Evy underwent surgical removal of her lower left lobe at Stanford Hospital. And she's now NED, no evidence of disease. She'll have follow-up screenings for at least five years but currently requires no chemotherapy or radiation.

"I know my case was kind of a fluke, but it still highlights the importance of early detection diagnosis. Lung cancer kills more than the other three deadliest cancers combined. We need to change that. We need to do whatever it takes to change that. I'm one of those rare people who has been on both sides, patient and caregiver. Neil was diagnosed at stage IV when he was sixty-three. If we'd found the cancer when he was sixty, he might still be alive today."

Her fervent advocacy for early detection led Evy to write an impassioned letter to Supreme Court justice and cancer survivor Ruth Bader Ginsburg.

"You are probably aware," she wrote in one paragraph, "that in 2015 Medicare approved coverage of low dose lung cancer CT screening for a high-risk population ages 55–77 who currently smoke or have quit within the past fifteen years and had smoked an average of one pack a day for thirty years. Based on this criteria, you, I and thousands more do not qualify for screening…but imagine if, like testing for colon, breast and prostate cancer at a certain age, all Americans were tested for lung cancer? How many lives and how much money would be saved in the long run? Discovering lung cancer should NOT be due to accidentally breaking a rib, as you did, or luckily reading a newspaper article, as I did."

I asked her if Justice Ginsburg ever responded.

"No," Evy said, "but I so hope that someday soon a well-known lung cancer survivor, or relative of one, will come out and help us in fighting this disease that's handicapped by misconceptions and still carries great stigma. Anyone can get lung cancer, just like Neil and I did."

I ask her what she would tell her high school students about her experience, if she were still in the classroom.

"I'd tell them the road is long, full of twists and turns, hooks and swerves. That's what life is. You're not in charge of where the road's going to turn next. Sure, we can choose which route to follow, but life always throws up detours on the way. So don't be afraid to peek around the next bend to see what's coming. You don't expect it and don't want something bad, yet even something bad can turn into a positive experience. Some of the best things in my life have come as a result of my cancer: the friends and people I've met, all the rewarding work I've done. The things that sometimes don't look so wonderful can offer wonderful opportunities. Cancer opens up a world to you that you never could have imagined. I think that's what any life-threatening illness will do."

Evy stops. I think she's finished, but then she continues, still very much back in high school teacher mode.

"If you think back to history class, you may recall that World War II was fought in three major theaters: European, Pacific Asian, and African-Middle Eastern. It turns out fighting cancer is a lot like a world war. I found this out when Neil was diagnosed with lung cancer that had spread to his brain, and I've come to think of the body as the world mapped out into different theaters, with campaigns launched in each to fight the enemy, which in this case is lung cancer."

I start to respond, but Evy isn't finished yet.

"Lori Gottlieb, the bestselling author, therapist, and speaker, tells a story about a young pregnant woman who lost her baby to a miscarriage. She was understandably devastated, didn't know how she could go on, until her friend sent her a parable: A woman has waited her whole life to go to Italy. It's her dream, and she's finally on board the plane that's going to take her there. But the plane gets rerouted, ends up in Holland, and she's devastated. But then she figures there must be wonderful things to see in Holland as well. *Maybe*, she thinks, *I can see the tulips*. That's the way Neil was and the way I want to be. I say to myself, 'Welcome to Holland, Evy.'"

Cancer might have slowed Neil Schiffman down, but it never stopped him. He was a fervent cyclist, but when he couldn't bike anymore, he took up hiking. I recall from his visits to the Living Room how he was always swapping one avocation for another, his cancer winning some of the battles while he was focused on winning the war. His last trip before a final downturn was to his fiftieth high school reunion at Boston Latin in his and Evy's native Massachusetts. It turned out to be the last time he would see his closest childhood friends.

I glance at Evy across the bench on the sidewalk outside the restaurant and see lung cancer at its most insidious, robbing a couple of the next twenty years packed with experiences and memories that will never be now. She deserved better; all those who've lost a loved one to any cancer deserve better. Neil remains a vital part of Evy's life, her memories of him so full and rich. The problem is there will be no more of those, and the memories that come now will be made without him. Too often that reality stokes dark moments for Evy, the kind of memories that are painful to hold.

"I remember early on how Neil had so much edema, we had to buy slippers that were three sizes bigger so that he could fit his swollen feet into them. He'd been diagnosed a few weeks before our wedding anniversary, and our tradition was to do something physical on that day: take a walk, a hike, or a bike ride. That year we decided to walk on a short, flat trail in Huddart Park not far from our home. All I could think of the whole time was whether this might be the last anniversary we ever got to celebrate after almost forty years of marriage. It turned out we had a few more together, but I'll always remember renting a hospital bed to put in our bedroom when we finally knew the end was near. I'd gaze at him and see someone who'd been an Ironman competitor looking like a survivor from a concentration camp."

Yet even that thought sparks another, more positive memory for Evy.

"I remember how down I was during that walk at Huddart Park, when the cell phone rang with a call from Stanford telling us that we had an appointment to see the oncologist we'd been trying desperately to get in to see. Her office told us we could come in that very afternoon. The strange thing was cell service was terrible on that trail, but that call somehow got through when we so needed some good news. I look back at the call as an anniversary gift."

The hostess appears to tell us our table is ready. We rise from the bench, but Evy isn't ready to go inside yet.

"When you lose someone you've been with your whole adult life," she reflects, "you have to come to grips with that every single day. You think about the things you'd planned out that you're not going to do. At the supermarket, you look at your cart and the things he used to pick up when you shopped together aren't there. You see two people holding hands and think that you don't have anyone to hold hands with anymore."

Evy was Neil's caregiver, and now she plays that same role with the couple's aging dog.

"Cubby keeps me going," she says, smiling. "What would he do if I wasn't there to take care of him?"

She's making a great point. Caregivers like Evy suffer a double loss when they lose someone like Neil. The person whom you always relied on to split responsibilities can no longer do them.

"You lose your copilot," as Evy says.

A mountain of tasks is thrust upon caregivers, to the point that they are living the other person's life more than their own. The priorities of the person they're caring for become their priorities, something that's all-consuming. When they lose their Neil, there's this incredible void and it's almost like they've forgotten how to fill it. Having focused on someone else's life for so long, they need to learn how to live their own again. You come home to the house you shared for so long and the emptiness is palpable, the quiet disconcerting. Where the sounds associated with two people once filled the house, there is only one. I've known caregivers who looked for excuses not to go home when their Neil passed. Maybe Evy's own cancer has filled that void for her a bit. Maybe it has even drawn her closer to Neil in his absence.

"I think what I'm doing now is the most important work I've ever done," she says as we finally start moving toward the restaurant entrance. "Teachers all want to believe they have the opportunity to change lives. I know what I'm doing now is changing lives."

I think about how caregivers deal with filling the void in the aftermath of losing a loved one and realize Evy just encapsulated her recipe for managing just that by confronting head-on the disease that so changed her life.

"Lung cancer is the leading cancer killer among women in the US, surpassing breast cancer in 1987," Evy's letter to Justice Ginsburg says. "It's estimated that in 2018 more than 70,000 American women died of lung cancer: 193 women every day, 8 per hour, one death every 7 minutes. During the past 39 years, the lung cancer death rate has fallen 29% among men while increasing 102% among women. I am joining with other patients to form an 'Early Detection Advocacy Group' to educate and advocate for screening to save lives. We would be honored if you would accept our invitation to be among our first members. Both Bonnie Addario and I would welcome the opportunity to travel to Washington, D.C. to talk with you and to thank you for helping us to achieve our goal of making lung cancer (and all cancers) a chronically managed, survivable disease, like AIDS, diabetes and so many other diseases. Through patients mobilizing we can save lives by educating the public, increasing research finding, and sounding the alarm that lung cancer is, amazingly, 29% of all cancers. Together we can change this!"

Although she never heard back before Justice Ginsburg's passing, Evy says she wasn't really expecting to. It was a letter she needed to write and she isn't about to stop writing them to anyone she feels can serve our cause.

As we head toward our table, Evy says, "I want to know that I have used my time and my capabilities to the max helping others, just like Neil did."

The previous chapter on Evy and Neil Schiffman highlights how caregivers play a vital role in lung cancer treatment for their loved ones—caregivers like Lorraine Kerz, who cared for her twenty-nine-year-old son Silas when he contracted lung cancer and became a fierce advocate in the wake of his death to honor Silas's memory. In June 2019, she gave this interview to the Lung Cancer Alliance about her experience.

1. Tell us a bit about yourself and your personal connection with lung cancer. Why does lung cancer advocacy matter to you?

My son Silas (Sy) was four days shy of his twenty-ninth birthday when he went to the ER because he was in too much pain to get out of bed on his own. He thought that he had pinched a nerve in his neck but was diagnosed with stage IV lung cancer that had metastasized to his bones. Silas went through chemotherapy, radiation, and two surgeries in the eight months after his diagnosis before he passed on. It was devastating to watch my son face his own mortality at such a young age, and yet he never once asked, "Why me?" He lived those months to the absolute fullest and handled his illness with a lot of determination, humor, and gratitude toward those around him.

Watching Silas decline and then losing him has been the hardest thing I have ever gone through; he was so young and excited about life. When Silas was sick, we came to realize that lung cancer is highly stigmatized and began talking about working toward ending the stigma. I made a promise to him that I would do whatever I could to be a part of creating change. I had hoped that somehow we would get a miracle and Sy's voice would be in the forefront of lung cancer advocacy. After he passed, I knew that as part of honoring my son's memory, I would do whatever I could to educate others and advocate for change in the world of lung cancer.

2. How do you feel that sharing your story has made an impact? Does one person have the power to make a difference?

I think that Sy's story is powerful. He was young, charismatic, and driven, with his entire adult life ahead of him until lung cancer struck. He was what I would call a warrior—battling his cancer with tenacity, humor, and a fierce passion for life. He had a way of being able to feel the terror of bad news and yet find something delightful to focus on a day later and the persistence to carry forward even during the darkest of times. His life affected those around him; not only his family and friends but also the medical team (doctors, nurses, his social worker, and orthopedic surgeon) that cared for him.

It is my responsibility to tell his story now that he is no longer here to tell it himself, and I do believe that it makes a difference. Change takes time, and with lung cancer it can't be fast enough, but I see the positive changes that have taken place over the past eleven years with research providing new treatments and new information on lung cancer, as well as low-dose CT scans now being used for early detection—giving people with lung cancer a better chance for survival. It's long overdue, and there is certainly much more to be done. "It takes a village," as the saying goes, and it is an honor to be part of that "village" for change.

3. How has your involvement in lung cancer advocacy led to meaningful connections with others in the community?

I have met so many wonderful people within the lung cancer community. We have laughed and cried and worried together; celebrated good news and mourned the setbacks and losses. We are a group of people who have had our lives changed forever through something we had no control over. There is an understanding within that group that is unique to those of us who are living with this reality.

I met my partner, Ken, through the tragedy of lung cancer loss. Ken lost his wife, Sheila, to lung cancer, and we met at a Lung Cancer

Alliance summit. We bring a unique understanding into our relation-ship that would be difficult for most others who have not lived with this type of loss to get. We also bring a lot of joy and lightness into each other's lives, as we both understand how precious life is and how it can change in a moment's time.

4. If you could give one piece of advice to someone who wants to get involved as a lung cancer advocate, what would it be?

Recognize that whatever you have to offer, it is worth getting involved. There is support out there and many different ways to become involved in advocacy. I didn't want to see other parents have to watch their child take their last breath because progress had not been made. It gave me the courage to take that first step and to keep going with it over the past eleven years since losing Silas.

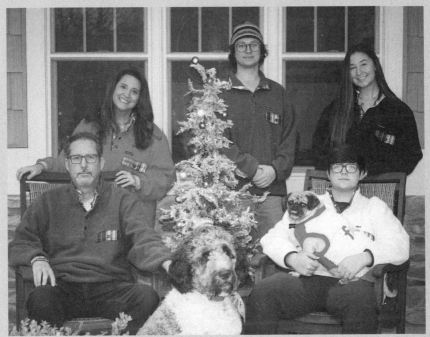

Michael McCarty and family, Christmas 2020

11

Michael McCarty

In October of 2018, then six-year lung cancer survivor Michael McCarty was the subject of a profile for a St. Joseph Mercy Health System blog under the heading BE REMARKABLE, something he finds oddly ironic.

"Because I don't see myself as remarkable," Michael tells me eighteen months later. "People will say, 'Oh, you're so strong, so amazing,' and I tell them, no, I'm just human. People see me that way because to them I'm unique. They all have a story to tell of someone they've lost. They'll say, 'I heard you had lung cancer. It killed my aunt in six months.' And they marvel that someone is standing in front of them with the same disease that took their loved one. That makes me remarkable to them. But I interact with people like me all the time. There's more than just one unicorn out there. And if we do things right, there'll be lots more unicorns in the not so distant future."

I spoke to Michael over the phone, having called him at his office on a beautiful Friday afternoon in Michigan, weather mirroring what was outside my window in the San Francisco Bay Area. His mood was reflective, since this now seven-year lung cancer survivor had just witnessed his daughter, who was eleven at the time of his diagnosis, graduate from high school—something he never thought he would see.

"When I was diagnosed, there wasn't even a targeted therapy approved yet for ALK-positive patients and I was given eighteen months to live. Now we have five approved treatments, with more trials in progress. We're making real progress toward turning lung cancer from a terminal disease into a chronic one."

Michael was diagnosed in September 2012 with non-small cell lung cancer, a type of cancer that occurs mainly in current or former smokers. As he would soon learn, it's also the most common type of lung cancer seen in nonsmokers like him. It was a stage IIIB diagnosis, borderline stage IV, and the cancer was progressing quickly, ravaging his body.

"It was a hot day in early August 2012, and I was out running when I ran into some friends on the road and decided to join them," he wrote in a November 2014 blog post for the Lung Cancer Alliance. "I knew for the last several months that my running pace was off and my workouts were less than to be desired, but I kept thinking I was simply lacking motivation after running a half marathon earlier in the summer. As the four of us started off, I called on my body to push itself and set a healthy pace, but my body had no answer and its silent stubbornness left me frustrated. And after falling behind the group, I stopped running and started walking. My friends were kind and tried to reassure me that the heat was the cause. However, I knew better. And less than a week later, I felt a lymph node start to pop out on the right side just above my clavicle."

Because Michael wasn't a smoker, pretty much everything but lung cancer was considered as possible ailment. When a pulmonary specialist couldn't see him for eight weeks, he found a general surgeon who agreed to perform a biopsy.

"I'll never forget the day he called me into his office to tell me I had lung cancer and it was advanced. My wife and I left the doctor's office and we sat down in the first chairs we saw and I then pointed to the survival rate I had written down on a piece of paper and started to cry. And for the next month, I was lost in a fog of anxiety, fear, and anger as to why this was happening to me."

The surgeons told him his cancer was inoperable, but Michael was able to get into a trial being conducted at Houston's esteemed MD Anderson Cancer Center, where he also met an oncological-radiologist he calls "Dr. Hope" because of the unique protocol she came up with to treat him.

"At the stage I was diagnosed, and because of the number of tumors in my lungs, around my heart, including one wrapping itself around the pulmonary artery, I was told at MD Anderson that traditional radiation would have killed me within two years of treatment, if the cancer didn't. Ironically, Dr. Hope was two years old and living in Hiroshima during World War II when the bomb dropped. And she was left feeling that if radiation can destroy lives, maybe it can save lives too. The cancer was so pervasive through my entire thoracic region that she tried proton therapy [a type of particle therapy that uses a beam of protons to irradiate diseased tissue] on me, thirty-eight treatments, in combination with weekly chemotherapy, that bought me the time I needed. You see, when I was diagnosed, doctors didn't find a treatable mutation."

After his initial treatment, he was declared NED, no evidence of disease, which lasted for eleven months until the cancer came back with a vengeance, and in this case that cliché is warranted.

"I had pleural effusion, pericardial effusion, a nine-centimeter mass in the right upper lobe, nodules on the left lung, cancerous tumor on the spine, cancerous lesions in the eyes, many lymph nodes lighting up throughout my chest, and two lymph nodes pushing against my esophagus preventing me from eating. Even though I made it home from the hospital, I was in tremendous pain, on oxygen twenty-four/ seven, and during a short month's time I lost forty pounds. My local oncologist gave me months to live as the cancer was spreading and spreading quickly. However, I was tested for the second time for the

ALK mutation. This time, I unequivocally tested positive for the ALK fusion. I was placed on a targeted therapy and within a week, my pain was gone, I was off oxygen, and I felt well enough to get into the gym (although only for a very light workout). Within weeks, my family and I were vacationing in the Keys giving God praise for what we call the 'Magic Pill.'"

And, for him, giving credit to God is more than just lip service.

"What I call the roar of diagnosis really knocked me off-kilter. For an individual who'd gone through life so certain about who he was and where he was headed, it was beyond unsettling. For days I sat with my Bible right in front of me, basically screaming, 'Why me? Why me, Lord?' It was anger, it was visceral. The only place I could go was to that little book I'd pushed away years before.

"One morning I got a call at the crack of a dawn from an executive in the company where I work telling me his father-in-law wanted to meet me for breakfast. So I met up at a Tim Hortons with a man I came to call 'Clarence,' after the angel in the great film *It's a Wonderful Life*. Clarence gave me one verse from the Bible, a psalm actually about being renewed. And I've been on a journey of Christian faith ever since. And that faith has sustained me through all the setbacks I've experienced, what I like to call detours. When I take one of these detours, the strength of God is what has sustained me for seven years now. I come to work every day, secure in the notion I'm pursuing whatever plan God has for me. Things that are within my control, I go out and control. Things that are outside my control, I accept that and lean on God's strength. That's how I've been able to get past 'Why me?' and go on, just decide to proceed. Without my faith, I don't know if I could have done that."

And Michael has practiced what he preaches—literally.

"In 2014, when my cancer returned after an eleven-month remission, I was told I had less than six months to live. Thanks to the targeted therapy I was given, six weeks later I was playing volleyball with my kids on the beach in Key West. We're walking down the street, watching the drunks, jugglers, and bicyclists, and there's this woman on the sidewalk faking an orgasm. My eleven-year-old daughter stops and asks me what that woman was doing. And I was so glad to be there in that crazy, priceless moment, there for my daughter to ask that question, because who else was she going to ask? I started thinking maybe there are other questions I could answer, that maybe I had another purpose to serve. So I got heavily involved in lung cancer advocacy, engaging people about my story to help them in their journey. I mentored patients, spoke publicly, and formed relationships with people I ended up growing amazingly close to, though, sadly, not all of them are still with us."

Michael credits any number of the relationships he's fostered as the reason why he's alive today and cites one to me in particular.

"I got to know this amazing lung cancer nurse, Lara Blair, who was a lung cancer survivor herself. I had first encountered Lara while attending a lung cancer advocacy outreach in Washington, DC, put on by Lung Cancer Alliance. She later asked me to speak at her hospital, St. Joseph Mercy. Shortly after speaking at St. Joe's, I started down an especially bad detour and ended up in my local hospital with my lungs full of fluid. I was pretty bad off, and I realized that if I stayed in my local hospital, I would die. My wife asked me where I wanted to go. I said St. Joe's. The next question was how to get there. My last memory before going unconscious was telling her to get in touch with Lara.

"My wife managed to get a message to Lara through Facebook, who was in a bed at that very hospital, having suffered a bad reaction to medicine after having a double knee replacement. She pushed all the right buttons and reached out to the right people, forcing the issue before she literally passed out. Thanks to Lara I got to St. Joe's, but unfortunately by the time I got there I needed a tracheotomy to be able to breathe. This prevented me from taking a new groundbreaking drug orally that had just gotten approved in the US. However, my new oncologist reached out to the manufacturer of the therapy in Japan and came up with a way where I could receive the medication through a tube in my stomach. I went from not being expected to make it through the night to leaving the hospital thirty days later."

So much of Michael's experience echoes that of other lung cancer patients I've met. He's struck up relationships that have been vital to his survival, and he's become his own best advocate, never taking no for an answer, never giving up. He's educated himself on the disease enough to know all the right questions to ask and the answers not to accept. He stresses how living with cancer has left him more in tune with his body and more aware of his limitations, but not in a discouraging way.

"When I gave my testimony at church, I actually said I look at cancer as a gift. People look at me in a strange way when I say that, but I'm a better husband, a better father, and a better employee now. I had been a very aggressive attorney, arrogant. At the time of my diagnosis, I was doing these big deals. I traveled around on fancy planes wearing custom suits, but something like cancer brings you back down to earth. You start focusing on what matters, instead of missing my kids' birthdays and showing up as a resident in my own home. Expecting love but not dispensing it."

If you win the rat race, you're still a rat, right?

"One of the things you think about when you have a terminal disease is that you've been prioritizing the wrong things. I've been fortunate to learn those lessons at the age of forty-three when I was diagnosed and now to have lived long enough to enjoy their fruits. So my perspective hasn't just changed, it's gotten better."

Well, not entirely.

"There are things I struggle with, like the old 'hunting and gathering' thing of working to provide because I'm my family's sole provider. I do what I do every day at this point because I need to. I really don't want to work until I die, but that's probably the reality. My wife and I were so looking forward to our senior years to do the things we never had time for. That still might be the case, but it's also possible that I won't get to that moment I'd long wished for, might not be able to enjoy those years with her. I struggle with that and work as hard as I can through everything, so at the very least my wife can enjoy her senior years, even if I'm not there with her."

So often when patients talk about the scourge of lung cancer, any cancer really, that becomes a dominant theme. How more than anything the disease has robbed them of their future, at least the certainty of it. Michael's passionate about a lot of things, not the least of which is the need to have repeat biopsies over the course of treatment as the cancer evolves, mutates, and develops resistance to one treatment after another.

"When I was first diagnosed, there was one targeted therapy drug. Now there are four, five actually, with more on the way. How do doctors know the best sequence of those drugs to follow? Well, they really don't after the first one they administered stops working. The only way to know the best one to use next is to have another biopsy to determine which of the remaining drugs out there is the right fit for you. Which biomarkers are indicated in each particular progression. And by collecting and sharing this data, we can better study and learn how cancer becomes resistant.

"One of the other things we're working on is to get more local, community-based hospitals to do the initial biomarker testing. Too many of them are not doing the genomic testing to determine if there's a targeted therapy that's right, which means the patient isn't getting the highest quality of treatment from the start. We've learned so much since my initial diagnosis, especially in the area of onco [oncological] gene-driven cancer. For instance, ALK-positive lung cancer is a protein-addictive cancer. Take the protein away and the cancer can't survive, so the therapies of today work by starving the cancer. Some patients get only a fractional response. I'm blessed because I've gotten one hundred percent. I'm on a drug now that was expected to work for nine months, and I'm now in my thirty-eighth month of treatment on it. There are times too when a drug that's stopped working in the past might start working again, thanks to the sub-mutations in a patient's particular cancer. Rare, but you just never know, and you never will until you ask all the questions and exhaust all the possibilities."

But one thing we do know about Michael McCarty is that he will remain a fierce advocate in the battle against lung cancer, both for himself and just as much for the others getting diagnosed in his wake. I was struck by something he said in a blog he'd written: "We should all push our doctors for quality of life." I ask him what he meant by that, since I'd never seen it put that way before.

"Doctors often focus on one thing: your scans. So they're treating the scans and not the person. You might say to them, 'Doctor, I'm not sleeping. I'm in pain. Let's focus on that instead of just the scans.' Or 'Great, I'm cancer-free, you might say, but there's no quality to my life. I'm too sick and weak to get out of the bed. Do we need to back off a dose of a drug I'm taking?' Patients need to engage their doctor in that kind of conversation to encourage him or her to treat the total person."

The roller coaster ride that defines cancer is a constant balance of highs and lows, ups and downs. Michael has been through more than his share of both and considers himself ever so fortunate that, so far anyway, every low has been matched by a high. And what I take from our conversation is how well he's coped with the lows. It feels like he's earned those highs, doesn't it? And more than anything, that's the quality that defines lung cancer patients: their relentless refusal to give up, to surrender to the disease that's done its utmost to hold them hostage, to steal their lives along with their health. Patients like Michael refuse to buckle under lung cancer's weight and burden. That makes them special. That defines the entire nature of their struggle.

"The first thing I tell recently diagnosed patients," Michael tells me, "is make sure to have a caregiver go with you to all appointments. Second, get the biomarker testing, and, third, be your own advocate. It's important to be there for new patients because sometimes what they need more than anything else is to engage with someone who's been through the same thing. And if I can survive this long, I tell them, so can they."

To mark his six-year "cancer-versary," Michael was a patient speaker at the annual Shine a Light on Lung Cancer event to showcase his perspective and his story.

"That initial diagnosis is like the sound of a train coming right at you down the track, so loud and overwhelming that you shut down. You need someone there with you, to hold your hand both figuratively and literally. Sometimes as a patient you have to steer your doctor in the right direction. I use myself as an example because, since I'm so knowledgeable about my disease, I have a better relationship with my doctor to the point that he calls me when he hears of something new coming out. We engage on that level. It's a matter, I like to say, of keeping the ball in the air—that's the objective. It's going to come down, maybe multiple times through the course of treatment, but the idea is to get the ball up again no matter what. Because as long as the ball's in the air, you're alive."

We talk about the incredible advances made in lung cancer treatment over the course of Michael's experience with the disease, opening the door to pose my favorite question: What are your three wishes for the future?

"So I'm rubbing the magic lamp and waiting for the genie to pop out. Okay, number one would be cure cancer—all cancer, not just lung cancer. My second wish would be to see my youngest son graduate high school. I got to watch my first two, and I'd love to see him graduate too. But he's only going into his freshman year, and we have a long way to go. My third wish would be to grow old with my wife, so we can hang out and do all the stuff we used to do before life took over. And to watch her smile and laugh our way to the end."

One of the most inspiring things in the world of lung cancer is the way relatives and caregivers respond upon losing a loved one. While not necessarily typical, this story of John Matthews has come to define the spirit and resilience of those who've lost a piece of their life to the disease. John can never get his mother back, but he's doing everything in his power to ensure others don't lose theirs.

ONE MAN'S 3,400-MILE RIDE TO END LUNG CANCER

That's the title of a superb post by Christine Donato on the SAP (Systems, Applications & Products in Data Processing) blog, referring to her friend and colleague John Matthews, who covered 3,400 miles riding his bike from Philadelphia to my home in the Bay Area. He did that in honor of his mother, Kathleen.

"John's initiative, 'Ride Hard Breathe Easy,'" Christine wrote for the blog, "is purposed to change the course of lung cancer—a cause to which John has wholly dedicated himself for the past [seven] years."

Kathleen had finally lost her six-year battle with the disease in 2017, leaving behind six children and nineteen grandchildren. John had no choice but to accept his mother's passing, though not its cause. He felt he had to do something to at least draw attention to the disease that had so changed his life. Even before setting out on his cross-country bike ride, John had left his mark.

"As each year passed," Christine Donato wrote, "John's family became more and more involved in raising funds to end lung cancer. John's running team, 'Kathleen's Krew,' raises the most money of any team at the BJALCF Philadelphia 5K every single year. In 2016 the team brought in a staggering $22,000."

The Bonnie J. Addario Lung Cancer Foundation offered significant support to John to make his trek possible. Still more support came from the Lung Cancer Foundation, the Lung Cancer Alliance, Lung Cancer Initiative, Adventure Cycling Association, and Guy's Bicycles.

I never cease to be impressed, if not amazed, by the commitment of people like John who refuse to knuckle under to the toll lung cancer takes on their families. They turn untimely death of a loved one into the preservation of future lives, and tragedy into inspiration. They are warriors on the same front in the war I've dedicated my life to fighting and that I know we will ultimately prevail in, thanks to them.

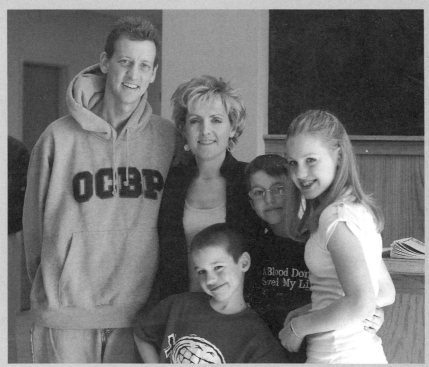

Lara pictured with her family just after her lung cancer diagnosis in 2007. Her husband Bill was receiving treatment for his own cancer at the time.

12

Lara Blair

My advice to anyone experiencing a lung cancer diagnosis? Know that it is not a death sentence and that for every type of cancer at every stage there are people who LIVE! Why shouldn't that be YOU? Be receptive to kindness and help when it is offered, and reach out when you need support.

—From a post by Lara Blair on the Lung Cancer Alliance blog

Imagine caring for your husband, who's suffering from a rare malignant thymoma.

Imagine being diagnosed with lung cancer yourself in the midst of all that.

"It was the hardest year of my life," Lara Blair wrote in a post on the Lung Cancer Alliance blog that led me to reach out to her, "but in many respects, it was also the best. Our family was surrounded and supported by many friends, parents, and other family members, coworkers, our kids' school teachers, fellow churchgoers, and medical team members. The outpouring of kindness and generosity gave our family strength that we could never have had on our own. To be on the receiving end of so much love and kindness was awe-inspiring, and we are forever grateful."

Lara's husband, Bill, died in 2012, and his funeral remains a blur in Lara's memory.

"It was surreal, one of those days like the day they tell you that you have cancer. I felt detached, like I was watching everything from the outside. It was like I was on a merry-go-round that was standing still while the rest of the world was rotating around it."

But she's alive and thriving today, twelve years after her initial diagnosis along a journey filled with changes and challenges she's risen to on every occasion.

"I never imagined lung cancer could change my life in so many good ways, change me as a person in ways I could never have imagined," she says, summing up that twelve-year journey. "I only wish I knew back then what I know now."

So let's go back to then, back to 2007.

"I suddenly developed a dry, hacking cough," Lara wrote in that same Lung Cancer Alliance post from September 2017. "In the preceding months I had lost some weight but had attributed it to the stress of supporting our family through the challenges of Bill's cancer treatment, which had started nine months prior. When the X-ray showed an area of concern, it was impossible to think that lightning would strike twice, but indeed I did have lung cancer. A 6.5cm tumor attached to the back of my chest wall and one lymph node showing reactivity on a PET scan. What followed next was almost a year of chemo, radiation, surgery, and more chemo."

A year she calls the best she'd ever experienced, only it didn't necessarily start out that way.

"I don't know how to describe it. Bill was so young and I was so young, and neither of us had risk factors. It was overwhelming, truly. But we had a really close group of friends, and we had an overwhelming amount of support from our church family. We'd spent years developing these deep personal relations with people who turned out to be there for us at every turn, who supported us, not just in practical ways but also in spiritual ways. Our kids were able to sleep over with any number of friends within five miles of our house. My parents even rented out their condo so that they could move closer to us to be able to help. Bill was being treated with radiation at the time I was diagnosed, so somebody had to come and take him to his treatments. We had more drivers than you'd believe. You make these friendships to celebrate the joys in life, but our friends were there for us when life got hard too."

I was connected with Lara through Michael McCarty. She was the lung cancer nurse, you may recall, who had just had both knees replaced when he contacted her through his wife, literally from what almost became his deathbed.

"Michael was at a loss as to what he should do. A lot of surgeons would have seen his case and told him it was time to let go. But his wife fought for him, went to every possible length to help. And I was able to direct her to a surgeon and an oncologist who saved his life."

Lara stops there, and I can picture her smiling on the other end of the line.

"All because we sat next each other on an airplane."

They'd never met, until a Lung Cancer Alliance conference that Lara calls "one of the most rewarding things I've ever done." After their paths crossed briefly at the conference, she and Michael ended up seated next to each other on the flight back to Michigan.

"Coincidence?" Lara poses wryly. "I don't think so."

We've never met, but I feel I know her almost from the start of our conversation. I guess a good portion of that is due to the fact that we're both lung cancer survivors, part of an ever-growing club typified by the kind of positive attitude Lara wears on her sleeve like an armband. I continue to be struck that so many survivors, like Lara, proclaim their cancer to be one of the best things that ever happened to them for the new perspective on life the experience has brought to them. And for lung cancer survivors, that new perspective provides a bond even tighter than blood. No one knows or can grasp the full extent of what we've been through, except another survivor. That's why so many survivors make themselves readily available to recently diagnosed patients to help guide them on a path that might otherwise swallow those patients up. It's like driving in the dark with your headlights off, unable to see what's straight ahead of you, never mind what's around the next curve. We provide that light for them and continue to shine it on each other in conversations like the one I'm having with Lara now.

To that point, I ask her to talk about the effect on their young children of having both parents suffering from cancer at the same time.

"Let's see, my kids were in eighth, sixth, and first grade when I was diagnosed. They were already watching their dad go through cancer—Bill was diagnosed nine months earlier—and now they had to watch their mom go through it. So I was determined to be strong, not to give up. The chemo they gave me made my hair fall out, and I got these wigs, five or six of them, each a different color. Before my hair even fell out, I dyed one of them this shocking pink. I wanted to do everything I could to change the equation. I didn't want this sense of despair to hang over everything. I didn't want people looking at me like that. I wanted us all to love the life we had and learn to laugh, really lean into our sense of humor.

"It's interesting how kids cope, though. There was this time during my chemo I got horrifically sick, so sick especially after this big surgery that I pretty much spent an entire summer in the hospital. Friends brought our youngest, Jeff, in to see me a few times. He's not a crier and always asked these mature, open-ended questions. But there was this one day he came to visit after his dad had thrown out his Sponge-Bob toothbrush that was just old and gross. He was heartbroken. And whenever he'd get really down or upset or hurt, he'd go back to talking about missing his toothbrush. So eleven years later I went on eBay and found him another, a replacement."

But eBay, of course, couldn't replace his mother. And the treatment she received assured that he didn't have to. Just as Bill was losing his battle with that malignant thymoma in 2012, she was beginning her recovery. Unlike many of the people you've met and will meet in these pages of our literary Living Room, Lara's particular form of lung cancer back then didn't qualify her for any of the cutting-edge targeted or immunotherapies.

She'd built a career over eighteen years working as a nurse in labor and delivery, a role she loved and excelled at. Lara literally spent her days working to bring new, healthy lives into the world, only to find herself facing death every day herself, first her husband's and then her own. And that experience paved the way for a new career when she went back to work.

"Soon after returning to my job working as a nurse in labor and delivery, the thoracic oncology team at my hospital asked me to join them in their multidisciplinary clinic as a nurse navigator for lung cancer patients. It was a great gift and an enormous privilege to be able to share what I had learned with patients going through a lung cancer diagnosis and treatment. And knowing how rare my recovery was, it gave a purpose to my survival.

"Becoming a navigator wasn't just about nursing, it was about becoming an advocate. I learned the power of advocacy and how impactful it can be when you speak not just with but also *for* patients. I'd get a call from a pulmonologist about a new patient and take things from there. I'd make up a folder for the patient containing all the information they needed when it came to testing, the financial end of things, palliative care, and set them up with the multidisciplinary clinic that would be determining their care. All the doctors and team members would gather in this small room to discuss that particular case to come up with a treatment plan. It was overwhelming for patients to be in that room, having so much thrown at them, and I did my best to make sense of it all for them. Sometimes I told them I was a cancer survivor, but I knew they were only going to remember about a third of what I said. I'd give them my cell phone number because that's what somebody had done for me when I was sick and I'd learned firsthand how important it was to have somebody they could go to directly, immediately. Someone who was always available to them. I wanted them to know there were a lot of treatment options available, that cancer wasn't a death sentence, that for every kind of cancer at every stage there's a population of patients who survive and do much better than expected."

I'm looking at a photo of Lara as we speak, picturing her with her three kids seven years younger than they are today. Mary's twenty-six now and is a first-grade teacher. Twenty-four-year-old Sam joined the navy and has graduated from the Naval War College in Newport, Rhode Island. At twenty, Jeff is still the youngest but far removed from the boy fretting over the loss of his beloved SpongeBob toothbrush. In the picture he's sporting a wide smile, with arms splayed over the shoulders of his mother and older sister. A brilliant family portrait that gives no indication of who's no longer there, only who still is.

"Jeff had an experience in high school that will stick in my mind forever. His dad had been gone for three years when a friend of his who had to leave school to be treated for lymphoma came back. 'David was at rehearsal tonight just to visit,' he told me. 'You know what's really weird? I could smell the chemo.' The smell was still stuck in his mind, even though it had been seven or eight years since his father had been treated with chemo. Kids absorb so much we're not aware of, and they don't necessarily articulate. I find myself always wondering how much more they absorb from the experience that will impact their lives, both good and bad."

Lara stops and starts again right away.

"There's a piece of advice I gave to a friend recently diagnosed with pancreatic cancer. His kids are about the same age as ours were when Bill died. When you're sick, when you're struggling to survive, you find yourself feeling sorry for your children, even guilty. So you tend to excuse things and reprioritize what you want your kids to be learning. That may be a very reasonable approach in the short term, but for us it was a six-year thing, and I know there were definitely some lessons our kids didn't learn because it just wasn't the most important thing to be doing at the time. Your kid might throw a tantrum, get into trouble at school, stomp up the stairs and slam the door, and your reaction might be something like, 'Hey, at least they're doing their homework.' They grow up in amazing ways that give them a unique kind of maturity, but sometimes they grow down too. The outcome is that there is learning that has to be done *later*, when they should be focused on other things, sometimes on their own (without their dad around), to make up for lessons that weren't taught because they were dealing with so much else. I felt badly about that as a parent and wished we had known at the time we were all going through it."

I remind Lara about how well her kids have all turned out. The proof, as they say, is in the pudding.

"What I've learned about lung cancer and cancer in general," she says, "is that attitude is a huge part of a successful outcome. But it's hard to maintain a good attitude in the face of so much adversity if you don't have support and help behind you from family and friends. Having friends and family gives you a reason to fight; otherwise, you risk developing a greater sense of hopelessness. You have the tendency to wonder, *What am I doing this for?* You need people to boost you up, something I was lucky enough to have. And the thing I enjoyed most about being a nurse navigator was that it's like the person who could get you backstage at a concert. And I worked with everyone! I could deal with the insurance company if they were refusing to authorize the PET scan. If one of my patients couldn't get in to see the doctor or department they wanted to for three weeks, I could walk their chart down the hall and get them in the next day. I loved making that kind of difference in their treatment and their lives.

"At one point I got involved in a list serve of small cell lung cancer survivors. People would post how long since they started treatment, and some were ten years removed from that point where their cancer was at its most pervasive stage. Others were five years, eight years. So I printed the list serve up, took it into that little conference room where the clinical patient meetings were held, and tacked it up on the wall.

Anytime we were gathered in that room, I'd direct everyone to that page to combat any negativity. I wanted all the doctors in that room to focus on that instead of a more negative outlook."

After Bill died, that role, always focusing on the positive, understandably became extremely taxing for Lara, given all that she'd experienced herself, something I can definitely relate to. So many lung cancer survivors have so much empathy, we end up absorbing the pain and heartache of others. For some, it's almost like reliving their own diagnosis and treatment—the ups and downs, the triumphs and disappointments, the good news and the bad. The sensation becomes visceral in its intensity, and sometimes it has the added effect of rekindling darker times in our own lives, almost like a physical flashback and a true shock to the system. But Lara didn't leave the world of cancer; she just redirected her efforts into another arena.

"I moved from being a nurse navigator into data collation and analysis, starting in the clinical registry arena. They wanted someone who knew this world, and I started working for my hospital's thoracic surgeons, who were participating in the Society of Thoracic Surgeons' General Thoracic Surgery Database, collecting data to provide them with tools to figure out where we needed to do better, where we were having problems. When I first started in the world of data, it was so boring compared to directly caring for people! But it turned out to be all about a commitment to patients, identifying problems so doctors could serve their cancer patients better. And I thought, *Hey, maybe data isn't so boring.*"

And working in data was also how she met a "wonderful man" named Gyula Sziraczky, president of ARMUS Corporation, a company he founded. According to his LinkedIn page, "ARMUS Corporation has always believed that accurate and clear interpretation of data will improve and transform cardiovascular interventions, and consequently improve patients' lives. Making this dream a reality motivates everything we do, and has guided ARMUS from our humble launch as a startup STS vendor to what we are today: a team of dedicated individuals constantly chasing excellence; producing technological innovations motivated by our clients and partners from regional initiatives and health systems."

They met at a conference where his company was supporting the state collaborative where Lara was working in data collection, a conference to which she had dreaded going. If she'd stayed home, though, her life would be in an entirely different place right now, almost surely one not as happy as where she finds herself today. But she has experienced her share of dark times amid the light that shines on her life, times she vividly remembers.

"The day after Bill was diagnosed, we were supposed to bring the kids to visit his family. He went to play golf, while my identity as a nurse took over in terms of 'we have this problem and need to deal with it.' When we were with his family, though, I realized how sick he looked, and I became terrified of him not making it, not being there. Most of the time when I broke down, I was alone—those were the worst times—which didn't happen too often, thankfully. But that continued after my own diagnosis through all the chemo and radiation treatments, when I'd wake up at four a.m. and find myself unable to go back to sleep. I'd go downstairs in the darkness and that's when I would cry. I'd sit there alone and stop thinking about all the reasons I had to live. I was struck by this panicky fear of death, that everything else was a distraction from the reality, that this was really happening to me and I wasn't going to be able to beat it. But those moments in the dark were also when I would pray, and I think that's what ultimately saved me.

"My relationship with God became so strong, I didn't feel alone anymore, even in the dark of those sleepless nights. Even in my worst moments, I felt the presence of God and I knew I had to live, I had to get well, and these are the things I have to do to make that happen. I had to live for my kids, live for my husband. My job was to take care of them, and I needed to get to work. Protect them from being sad, from anxiety, from fear. And when I focused on protecting them, I didn't feel that pain in the dark anymore, because I was more worried about theirs."

In some ways, when Lara describes lung cancer as one of the best things that ever happened to her in spite of those dark moments, she's talking about the second chance she found at love with a man she met, at least indirectly, as a result of contracting the disease as a nonsmoker with no other risk factors. Of course, that second chance at love followed the second chance at life she'd already been granted. She's remarried now and living in California, where Gyula's company is based, but her memories and love for her late husband made the move with her.

"The whole experience definitely brought Bill and me closer together because we had to take care of each other. It made our marriage really strong in an entirely different way. We became very focused on our faith, the good things in life, being grateful for what we had and not fixating on what we didn't. We learned never to take anything for granted."

Dr. David Gandara of the UC Davis Comprehensive Cancer Center is one of the foremost clinicians and researchers in the lung cancer field today. Dr. Gandara's research interests focus on developmental therapeutics of new anticancer agents as well as preclinical modeling and clinical research in lung cancer. He is the principal investigator on an early therapeutics award from the National Cancer Institute (NCI), where he leads an interdisciplinary team of clinical oncologists, pharmacologists, molecular biologists, and statisticians in developing new anticancer agents in a variety of novel drug classes. He also leads a multispecialty team in the Southwest Oncology Group (SWOG), an NCI-funded national clinical research organization, in studies related to improving therapies for lung cancer and developing predictive biomarkers of therapeutic efficacy. Here are his thoughts on the state of lung cancer treatment today.

Based on where we are today compared to five or ten years ago, where do you think we'll be or where might we be in ten years?

Never in the history of oncology have so many major treatment advances been seen over such a short period of time as for non-small cell lung cancer patients over the last five years.

What's the first thing you say to a just or recently diagnosed lung cancer patient?

I always start my conversation with a new lung cancer patient by saying, "How can I help you?" No matter who the patient is, young or old, man or woman, stage I or stage IV, these words resonate. This simple phrase is music to a new patient's ears.

What are the things about lung cancer everyone should know?

First and foremost, people need to know that anyone can get lung cancer, absolutely anyone! And lung cancer is so common that almost every family has been touched by it.

What surprises/impresses you most about the lung cancer patients you treat?

What impresses me most about the lung cancer patients I treat is their resilience. There is an inner strength which I have seen so often, which helps them rise above barriers and setbacks and to continue to enjoy every day despite facing a sometimes life-threatening illness.

What role have advocates played in lung cancer treatment?

Patient advocates are the heart and soul of the lung cancer community. They are a constant inspiration to doctors, nurses, and the rest of the lung cancer treatment team. And of course, you, Bonnie, are the best of the best. You speak with a unique perspective as a lung cancer survivor who has also dedicated your own time and resources to eliminating lung cancer. As has your entire family. There is nothing like it anywhere in cancer advocacy.

If you could change one thing about the way lung cancer is treated today, what would that be?

If I could make a wish come true, it would be that every single lung cancer patient worldwide today had access to all the resources and advances that are available, regardless of cost or where they live in the world. Now *that* would be a miracle worth seeing!

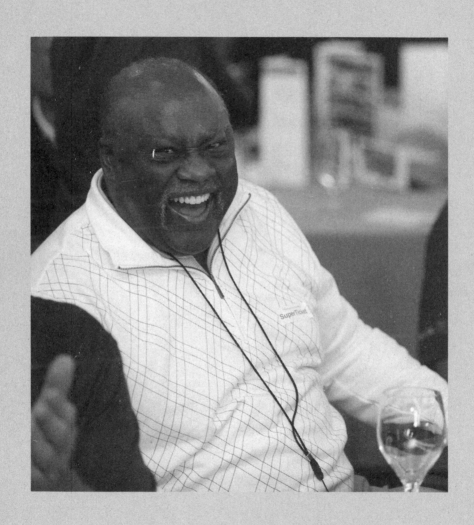

13

Hank "The Big Hug" Baskett

I first met Hank Baskett Jr. in 2012 at a golf tournament his son, Hank III, was sponsoring in support of lung cancer in conjunction with the Addario Lung Cancer Foundation. He wrapped me up in his huge arms, and right then and there, I nicknamed him "the Big Hug."

"Well," he said, grinning from ear to ear on a picture-perfect day at the Trump National Golf Club in Rancho Palos Verdes, California, over Memorial Day weekend in 2012, "I guess that makes you 'the Little Hug.'"

Hank was sixty-nine at the time but still looked every bit the part of the United States Air Force chief master sergeant whose deployments took him all over the world. He'd been diagnosed with lung cancer six months earlier, and I could tell right away by looking at him, particularly the swelling of his ankles and sickly pallor of his complexion, that he wasn't getting the treatment he needed. When the opportunity availed itself, I pulled him aside to tell him he had to see, just *had* to see, Dr. Ross Camidge at the renowned University of Colorado Cancer Center close to Hank's home in Clovis, New Mexico.

"The doctors diagnosed me with lung cancer," he says over the phone after we joke about our initial meeting seven years ago. I recall Hank's then two-year-old grandson, Hank IV, making his presence known on the links as well, though absent a golf club. "I gave it to God, and God is who brought me to you."

The physician who'd been treating Hank in Los Angeles from the spring of 2011 hadn't done the proper biomarker testing, not unusual at the time. But Dr. Camidge and his staff quickly determined that the Big Hug was eligible for a targeted therapy his original doctor had not made him aware of.

"I take one pill a day, one pill ever since. Seven years now. I went for a checkup in October of 2013 and they said to me, 'I don't see anything. Either it's gone or hiding very well.'"

"I told them, 'It's gone. God already took it.' But I don't fault those Los Angeles doctors for anything," he tells me over the phone from Clovis. "See, they kept me alive long enough to meet you and for you to get me to Dr. Camidge. That first time we met, I knew it was your heart speaking, and you captured my heart. You were like the Energizer Bunny. You wouldn't quit until I finally made that call. I flew back to New Mexico on a Sunday and called those folks on Monday, and they told me I already had an appointment to see the doctor because you'd already called and told them they had to see me right away. I'd hug you right now over the phone if I could. Feel it, I'm hugging you now!"

Dr. Camidge and the staff at the University of Colorado diagnosed Hank as having a type of lung cancer between A and B positive.

"'We are the people who discovered that strain of cancer,' they told me there, and they asked if they could put me in this study group. I told them if that helps find a cure for somebody else, go right ahead. Well, I hugged the nurse, I hugged the doctor, I hugged everybody. They were a blessing; you sending me there was a blessing."

It turned out that Hank had been treated for the wrong subset of the disease in Los Angeles, and Dr. Camidge found Hank to be a perfect candidate for a targeted therapy he can't remember the name of right now.

"I just got off the golf course," he tells me the evening we recently spoke to catch up six years after he began treatment. "Played eighteen holes."

I ask him how he was originally diagnosed.

"Being a veteran, I was getting this cough I'd had for two, three months checked out at the VA center across the border with Texas in Amarillo. I went there with my friend, a fellow vet named Bill McCormick. The doctor took X-rays, came back, and said, 'There's something I just don't like.' So he did an MRI and CT scan, came back again, and said, 'Like I thought, it's cancer in your lungs and it's bad.' He didn't tell me what stage it was or anything. I made another appointment to come back to get treated and drove home those few hundred miles with Bill Mac wondering how was I going to tell my wife, Judy. How do you tell a loved one you were just given a death sentence? Right there in the car, I said to myself, 'God's got it. Whatever You want, I'm ready.' So my wife was still at work when I got home, and as soon as she got back, she looked at me and said, 'What's wrong?' I told her, 'I got some news.' And when I told her, well, I never want to see that look on a person's face again.

"That Sunday, April 19, was Easter, and when I spoke to my son Hank III, he was at the Playboy Mansion with my two-year-old grandson Hank IV for Hugh Hefner's annual Easter Egg Hunt."

Hank III, I should mention, enjoyed a five-year career in the National Football League, playing for the Minnesota Vikings, Indianapolis Colts, and Philadelphia Eagles. He parlayed that experience into a stellar career in the entertainment industry after marrying Playboy model Kendra Wilkinson and came to consider Hefner something of a mentor when building his business and, especially, his brand.

"Next thing you know," the Big Hug continues, "Hugh Hefner got me set up with all these doctors. His assistant made all the calls and got me appointments with a primary, an oncologist, and a pulmonologist. Turned out I was stage IV, and they started me on treatment right away. That saved my life, kept me going long enough so God could get me to you and you could get me to the University of Colorado. That's the way He works, the way the world works. I tell people God let the cancer in there, so it must be for some reason. I didn't worry about it then, and I don't worry about it now. I don't even know that I have it. All I can say is that I'm glad it happened to me. I'd never want it to happen to anyone else, especially a child. I've done things in my life I'm not proud of and asked forgiveness. But what have little children or young people done to deserve this disease or any other? I think about those babies getting treated at places like St. Jude's, how they smile and laugh in spite of everything they're going through, and I think about people who complain when they stub their toe. I want to tell them to suck it up. Think about what you did in your life, and cry for those babies who never had a chance to do anything but still have the brightness in their eyes and can smile. Thinking about them, what have I got to complain about?"

I can picture him smiling as he says that, because the Big Hug is always smiling, the only exception being when we get around to discussing his work as director of Oasis Children's Advocacy Center, a safe house for abused children, a position he held for twenty-one years.

"I look at children's faces and I can tell when someone's hurting them. When I was diagnosed, I knew I had to keep working with the kids because I knew God wanted me to. When I'd interview a child concerning their abuse, I'd let Him do the interview through me because I didn't want to mess up with one of His precious little creatures. Working with those children gave me a new outlook on life. I dealt with families and directly with the abusers themselves, getting the police and social workers involved. Every time a child came to me, when I touched this child's life, it was for a reason. My problems were small compared to theirs. They were defenseless. They couldn't fight back against the guardians in their lives who hurt instead of protected them. When they left my office, I'd tell those kids to give it all to God. You are without sin, and He will take care of you."

I realize something in that moment. That this man who spent twenty-one years defending children against bullies faced the biggest bully of them all in lung cancer and stared it down. He stood up to it, just like he counseled the children in his office to stand up to their abusers because it's not their fault. They didn't ask to be hurt any more than Hank asked to get lung cancer.

"When I meet one of my grandkids' friends, I always say, 'May I have a handshake?' Because I want them to be empowered to make the decision to shake. It has to come from them, from the child. They have to feel they have the power, and not their abuser."

Just like Hank had the power and lung cancer didn't.

"Life is a choice. God gave us all free will. My father was an alco- holic who died of throat cancer from drinking that moonshine stuff. And people thought my daddy was like that so I'm going to be too. And it's true—I was a wild man as a youngster, putting that liquor down. It controlled me for several years, until I had to make a decision not to let it control me anymore. It's what I tell people: You are in control of you, even your cancer. You have a choice.

"I'm a big George Jones fan, the country and western singer, and he's got this song called 'Choices' that talks about voices helping you tell the difference between right and wrong. Everybody needs those voices, but you've got to listen to them when they talk to you.

"Once I was speaking to this kid who'd been abused, but he wouldn't talk to me no matter what angle I took. So I told him sometimes when you get a splinter in your hand or in your leg, you run home so your mommy can get the splinter out. It's gonna hurt, all that poking around with a needle before she squeezes that sucker out and it's gone, and you go, 'Ahhhhhh,' because you know she got it out of you. That's what I told this little boy: The splinter is just like when somebody does something bad to you. It's garbage, it's bad. You need to get it out of you before it gets into your blood and makes your whole body hurt. That's what we do with kids like that, because they come in for us to take the splinter out. I'm like the garbage can—I just suck it all in. And when one kid leaves, I'm gonna do the same thing with the next one who comes in. I'm gonna get rid of that splinter and give it to God. Then He's gonna take care of the rest."

In Hank's mind, the disease that nearly killed him is just another splinter. And he gave his lung cancer over to God.

"When you walk out of your house in the morning, you don't know who you're gonna meet or what's going on in that person's world. I'll go into the convenience store out here and say, 'How you doing this morning?' to the person standing in line next to me. 'That's a beautiful smile you've got there.' They always smile even wider when I say that, and that makes me glad I came in. If you can put a smile on every person's face, say just a kind word to them, you never know but you might have just saved that person's life. It could be at an airport when you're surrounded by strangers. That's the thing about life: you just never know."

Seventy-five now, Hank has retired from his work with abused children, something he wishes he'd started doing twenty years earlier. He doesn't know the exact number of kids he's helped, but he likes to believe, does believe, they've gone on to help others. They have that choice because the Big Hug gave it to them.

"I want to be like AT&T. You know, reach out and touch someone. That's what it's all about. Last year, Colorado University Medical Center had their first ever Survivors Summit, and they asked me to be a guest speaker. I don't know why they chose me. I said I'd do it, but I didn't know what I was going to say. So I told that audience, and it was big, that I don't worry about cancer. I'm so blessed it doesn't bother me. I'm gonna shut up and color because I know God will keep me between the lines. I refuse to let cancer beat me. It's been a long haul and I've enjoyed this ride and I'm gonna stay on it with every breath that God leaves in my body. If you're down, I'm gonna try to get you up. I'm gonna love you. But it all started with the Little Hug! Without the Little Hug I wouldn't be here now."

I can picture the Big Hug grinning thirteen hundred miles away. I'm grinning too, though I need to dab my eyes with a tissue.

"I had a checkup back in February and March, usual X-rays and scans. The nurse came in and pointed out a tumor on my lung, maybe two-point-five centimeters. She sounded worried, concerned. So I pointed to my shoulders on the X-rays and asked her, 'Do you see those hands right there?' She looked close but didn't notice anything. 'Look again,' I told her. When she said she still couldn't see anything, I gave her a big smile and said, 'That's because those are God's hands on my shoulders, right there on the X-ray."

That was the first I heard about this new tumor. Hank's been on the same drug for seven years and has gotten amazing results. When and if it stops working, there'll be another to take its place. At least that's the hope, because I can't imagine a world without the Big Hug, even though he doesn't seem bothered at all.

"I'm not worried 'cause I know He's got this. Maybe He's calling me home, telling me my time is almost up. Maybe it's because I'm strong enough, so I need to suck it up. Or maybe He let all this happen to me so I could be an inspiration to someone else. God's got the final say. He left me on this world to become a mentor to anybody who's going through something bad. So I can give them a spark and put a glow on their face, just let them know how precious life is. It's like a second career to me."

I think back again to that golf tournament, cohosted by his son Hank, where we first met in Rancho Palos Verdes. You meet Hank III and it's not hard to figure out whom he takes after. He's become even more heavily involved with lung cancer advocacy because he believes we're the reason his father is still alive. And because of Hank III's efforts, more people will survive to help others, paying it forward.

The circle of life, not the circle of death, to paraphrase the Big Hug

"Anyone that sits with him for just five minutes, they get up feeling better than when they sat down," Hank III told the *Clovis News Journal* in November 2013.

Hank III played pro football, but Hank IV, now nine years old, has opted for skates instead of cleats and the ice rink instead of the gridiron.

"He's like the wind," his grandfather reflects. "I watch him skate and I fall down. My son didn't like being one-upped by his boy, so now he's playing hockey in a men's league. He told me the other day he's never been in so much pain, that it was never this bad when he was playing in the NFL."

I ask Hank what advice he might give a recently diagnosed lung cancer patient.

"Number one thing is don't claim it. Don't run around saying, 'I have lung cancer.' Don't own it. You were diagnosed just like I was diagnosed, but I refuse to have lung cancer. It's in my body, but I don't own it, 'cause I gave it to God. And that's what you need to do too. Somebody asks if you have lung cancer, you tell them, 'No. I was diagnosed, but I don't have it. God's got it. God got me to that doctor in Colorado, got me to that pill, got me to the Little Hug!"

Hank's got three other kids, including two daughters from his first marriage. He and his wife, Judy, have been together now for thirty-three years.

I don't want our call to end. I wish I was in the same room with him so I could give the Big Hug a big hug and not let go. Because if I don't let go, he can't go anywhere. He'll always be there, a part of my life and so many others.

I ask Hank Baskett about the future, his plans, hopes, and wishes.

"Well, I don't have a bucket list because I've done all the things I wanted to. I love people, I just love people. I don't wish for nothing because I've got everything I want—well, maybe one wish: to see my grandkids grow up and become adults so I can have great-grandkids. I just thank God for this life I've had. He allowed me to be who I am. And you know what? If you shut up and color, He'll show up and guide you."

I think about that image and realize it sums up the essence of the Big Hug. It makes me think about all the people I've known who've lived their lives in black and white. Hank Baskett lives his life in color. Vibrant, brilliant color flashing like a kaleidoscope.

"People look at me and say, 'You don't look like you've got lung cancer.' I tell them that's because I don't let my spirits get down. Life's a choice, remember? And I choose joy. Every day you've got to walk out of your house with joy. If you don't have joy, go back to bed. I thank God for this life. He allowed me to be who I am, and I'm gonna keep on being me for as long as He lets me."

Dr. Louis Raez is chief of hematology-oncology and medical director at Memorial Cancer Institute/Memorial Healthcare System, one of the largest public health care systems in country. He also serves as president of FLASCO, the Florida Society of Clinical Oncology. Here are five questions I posed to him:

Based on where we are today with lung cancer treatment, compared to five or ten years ago, where do you think we'll be or where might we be in ten years?

We've just begun to cure people, and ten years from now a much larger number will be cured, thanks to advances in targeted therapies and immunotherapy. Precision medicine in general will allow us to identify genomic-based therapies that will lead to even more positive outcomes. We want to raise the survival rate of lung cancer from around twenty percent to one hundred, and our first goal toward that is to go from terminal disease to chronic and then to cure. That's a realistic expectation a decade from now.

What's the first thing you say to a recently diagnosed lung cancer patient?

That there is hope. It's natural for people to fall into despair on getting the news of their diagnosis. But we can treat you. We can keep you alive, even cure you.

What are some of your goals as president of FLASCO?

It starts with more funding for lung cancer. It's the top cancer killer there is, but funding is still woefully lagging between research funding for colon, breast, and prostate, among others. HIV was basically cured because of the amount of money that went to researching and developing the drugs that have generally eradicated it. We need that kind of commitment for lung cancer. We're also working with twelve industry partners in statewide projects that benefit cancer therapy outcomes for patients. For example, right now statewide we only screen about five percent of patients at risk of developing lung cancer, and we need to significantly increase that proportion. We have other projects regarding access to drugs, payment for drugs, and assuring that all patients get the best quality of care possible.

Can you talk about the importance of lung cancer screening?

The rate of people receiving colonoscopies has reached sixty percent, but it's still only five percent for lung cancer screening. Think about the high percentage of women who get screened for breast cancer. But lung cancer kills more than twice as many women every year, around eighty-five thousand, as breast cancer. Survival rates are much higher with breast cancer because breast cancer receives three times the amount of research dollars as lung. We could save far more women, and men, than we are right now with early screening.

What are your three wishes for the future of lung cancer treatment?

First, we need more funding. That would make a huge difference and it's what everything comes back to. Second, we have to learn more about tumors than we currently do, understand the course of their mutations better. Lung cancer is a smart cancer, and we need to get smarter to fight it. And my third wish is to make lung cancer something that can be cured. That may seem like a stretch, until you consider that twenty years ago precision medicine didn't even exist and the only available treatments were universal standards of radiation and, especially, chemo-therapy. Now we use a more disciplined approach to fight cancer. The breakthroughs have been incredible, but we need to see more.

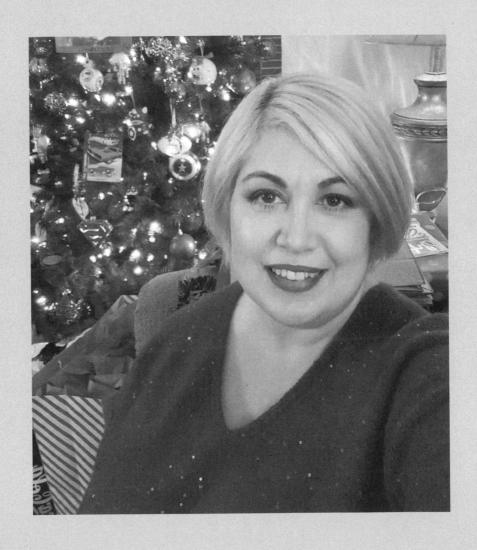

14

Juanita Segura

Someone sent me a video of a woman lifting weights, a lot of weight, an exercise that's called a dead lift. Having not noticed the tag from the link on Facebook, I wondered why they'd sent it to me.

BECAUSE SHE'S A LUNG CANCER SURVIVOR! the sender emailed me back.

I've never met Juanita Segura, a first-generation American born of a Puerto Rican mother and Mexican father who himself was an immigrant. But her particular story struck me as so impressive I had to reach out to her, via the same Facebook page on which the video was posted, and she reached back immediately.

"WOW! I would be honored to speak with you, Bonnie," she messaged me in response. "Thank you so much for this amazing opportunity to be included in your book."

That kind of graciousness and humility typifies this fifty-one-year-old mother and now grandmother. All lung cancer survivors display an incredible amount of strength, as much figurative as literal. But Juanita

195

has taken the literal to a whole new level, taking control of her cancer in the same manner with which she hoists kettlebells effortlessly overhead.

"If my little story can save two or three people," her initial message continued, "or give them hope so they can fight too, then I'm happy."

Juanita's story is anything but little. In the early summer of 2014, she developed a persistent wheeze. She thought nothing of it because she was a healthy eater, had never smoked, and was active in a training regimen known as CrossFit. I'd heard of CrossFit prior to hearing about Juanita, enough to know it was not something sick people did. The program is extremely strenuous and capable of testing the physical acumen and conditioning of even the most serious athletes. And the story of how she got into CrossFit in 2013, a little more than a year before her diagnosis, is something in itself.

"It was a really hard time for me. I'd lost my job and couldn't find another. We had to file for bankruptcy and I was really depressed. I heard through the grapevine that a friend of mine who ran a CrossFit gym needed a new website and business cards for promotion. So I told my husband, who works in that kind of business, and he made arrangements to go see my friend that Saturday. My friend told him to bring me so I could train while he was taking pictures for the website."

"I said, 'I'm not going to do that.'"

"'Well,'" my husband said, "'your friend said you better get your ass over there.'"

"I'd let myself go because I was so depressed over losing my job. I didn't even have any money to buy workout clothes, so I found some old capri pants and some stuff from my husband's closet and off I went."

CrossFit turned out to be entirely different from what Juanita had been expecting. Structured around the WOD, for Workout of the Day, it featured a mix of cardio exercises and weights with an emphasis on multiple repetitions instead of loading up the barbells. Juanita started push pressing with twenty-pound weights and picked things up fast. She noticed there were women in their sixties and seventies in the class.

She was already sweating and exhausted when her friend broke the news to her:

"That was just a warm-up."

Uh-oh, Juanita thought. *You mean I'm not done?*

Not even close. She had to keep repeating the exercises comprising the WOD until time stopped. She worked with kettlebells, then did push-ups and something called a box step-up, repeating the sequence over and over again.

"Are we done yet?" she kept asking.

"No, no, no," her friend told her.

"I complained the whole time. I was arguing with her. She told me to 'stop complaining and keep going.' So I did, and when we were finished, she told me I did great. And not only that, all these other people were watching me, shaking their heads. They couldn't believe it was the first time I'd ever done CrossFit."

But it was, and CrossFit went on to become a vital part of Juanita's life—before, during, and after her treatment for lung cancer.

"When we started doing dead lifts," Juanita says, referring to the exercise captured in that video that had served as our introduction, "my friend just kept adding weight and I kept doing the exercise. I don't know how much we got up to, but it was a lot. People were standing around watching, thinking *'Holy crap! This girl can lift!'* That gave me so much confidence."

Something she would desperately need as the months progressed after that persistent wheeze finally led to a doctor's visit in June 2014, a year almost to the day after she started CrossFit. She was diagnosed with asthma and prescribed an inhaler.

"I told him I don't have asthma, but he made me try the inhaler anyway."

Sure enough, the wheeze soon turned into a horrible cough. By October 2014, Juanita couldn't complete a sentence without coughing. A pulmonary specialist prescribed a steroid, but her condition continued to worsen.

"Not long before I started wheezing, I got certified as a CrossFit coach and was teaching the five a.m. class at my friend's gym. That was good, because I'd finish up and have the whole day in front of me to do other things. I never imagined that first day in the gym that CrossFit could become a career for me, but now I was thinking it could."

Not so fast. Juanita had a chest X-ray on which her pulmonologist noticed something on the right side that looked large and inflamed. He told her to come back the following week if the new medication he prescribed didn't make any difference. When it didn't, a subsequent CT scan revealed fluid under her lungs that could have been pneumonia until tissue samples taken during a bronchoscopy revealed something much worse.

"I knew it was something bad. A few days later, the doctor came in with a nurse and closed the door—that's always a bad sign. 'You tested positive for a malignancy,' he told me. My heart was racing so fast, I went numb. I couldn't comprehend what I'd just heard. It was like an out-of-body experience. All I could think of was my five kids and like the cancer had ended up in the wrong body or something. I asked the doctor what kind of cancer it was."

"'Lung cancer,'" he said.

"I looked at him and said, 'Dude, I don't even smoke.' I didn't even say 'doctor.' I called him 'dude.'"

"'You can get lung cancer even if you don't smoke,' he told me, and I'm thinking I'm never going to see my youngest daughter graduate high school or get married. I'm not going to be there for their college graduations. I had a one-year-old granddaughter. I wasn't ready to die."

When she started treatment at a Cancer Treatment Centers of America facility in Zion, Illinois, her oncologist told her she was the most fit and healthy patient he'd ever treated. Determined to beat her lung cancer, Juanita endured six weeks of chemotherapy and radiation. But she wasn't going to stop working out, doing CrossFit.

"I went on days when the side effects from the chemo weren't as bad, when I felt better. I didn't do the extreme workout, but I'd still lift.

There were days I couldn't go. But I always came back and paced myself. A guy who worked out there noticed I was losing weight because I didn't have any appetite, and he turned me on to protein shakes. I built myself back up, put the weight back on I'd lost. I even started coaching that five o'clock class again the same day my hair started growing back. That's when I knew I could beat this thing. I had to be strong for my kids. The worst thing about the whole experience was watching them break down. You know, I think CrossFit may have saved my life, that God had brought me to that gym for a reason."

But Juanita still had a very long road ahead, one that came with its share of detours, starting with the fact that it took six weeks of chemo and radiation to get her biomarker tests back.

"Turned out I was ALK positive," she laments, an edge creeping into her voice. "If they had come up with that result earlier, I could have avoided all the chemo and radiation, and I had a bad reaction to the radiation, which set me back even more. All I would have had to do was take this targeted pill—the chemo and radiation hadn't made any difference in my condition at all. The lung cancer was still there, still the same."

Upset and disappointed over her initial course of treatment, Juanita's sister made an appointment for her to go the Mayo Clinic in Minneapolis, where a nurse practitioner matter-of-factly spat out a stream of facts and statistics, the upshot of which Juanita was told she'd likely live only eighteen months in the wake of reviewing a PET scan the Mayo had ordered.

"I looked at her and said, 'Girl, you don't know the God that I serve.' My husband turned as red as a tomato, he was so shocked. But someone at the Mayo mentioned one of the best lung cancer specialists anywhere was right in my backyard at the University of Chicago. We flew home the next day and were at his office the day after."

Juanita stops and starts again right away, before I can probe that further.

"My dad died of cancer, and he went to the University of Chicago's hospital fifteen years ago. I'll never forget how well they treated my dad; they fought and fought and tried everything to save him. They gave him additional time so he could meet my daughter who's now fifteen. She was born, and my dad died a week later."

At the University of Chicago Comprehensive Care Center, Juanita began treatment with a protein kinase inhibitor. After about three months on the drug, the tumor in her lungs disappeared. However, her doctors discovered the cancer had spread to her liver. Juanita's treatment was switched to another drug, an ALK inhibitor for metastatic non-small cell lung cancer. Within three more months, the spots on her liver had shrunk significantly. She ended up going on *Dr. Phil* in 2016 to tell her story, piggybacking more than two dozen other interviews on top of that one while in New York.

"I want all cancer survivors, not only lung cancer survivors, to know there's hope," she said. "If my little story can save just a few people or give them hope so they can fight too, then I'm happy."

That story has a happy ending because of the care she found at the University of Chicago that neither Cancer Treatment Centers of America nor the Mayo Clinic had proved able to match. That's not necessarily a reflection on either of those facilities so much as a testament to Juanita and her husband's relentless quest to find the situation that was right for her. The fact that it turned out to be so close to home illustrates that, oftentimes with cancer, you don't have to travel great distances to get the best care. Different patients, different approaches, different protocols, and different settings can produce markedly different results. And one of my first recommendations for newly diagnosed patients is to find the care that's not only the most cutting edge and up to date, but also to seek out the situation that feels the most right to them. Juanita never really felt right at the first two venues but knew she'd found the right place as soon as she walked through the doors of the University of Chicago.

"And, five years later, I'm NED, no evidence of disease. I see Dr. Jyoti Patel now because my original doctor moved to California. I'll be on this pill for the rest of my life, but I don't think my cancer's ever coming back. Dr. Patel told me that and I almost fell off the chair. I want to still be doing CrossFit when I'm a hundred and two and meet my great-grandchildren, even my great-great-grandchildren! I want to be the oldest living lung cancer survivor in history, have a street named after me or maybe a hospital. I'm not going anywhere."

Speaking of CrossFit, not too long ago Juanita approached George, the owner of the CrossFit gym she'd been attending closer to home, and told him she wanted to open up her own gym.

"'My mother died of lung cancer,'" he told me, "'Go for it.' So I went from having lung cancer to opening my own gym. Who can beat that?"

Juanita wanted to attract more members, more people who might have been intimidated by the CrossFit name and brand, which conjured visions of Olympic-level athletes. So she called her new gym Redirect Fitness.

"People have been like, 'Wow! You have lung cancer and you're running a gym? Don't you get shortness of breath?' I tell them I'm fine. But I've gone through a lot, and all that chemo and radiation has done a number on my body, so I don't lift as heavy anymore. Sometimes my joints ache a little, but that's a small price to pay for being cancer-free.

"I just want to do for others what was done for me. This woman started training at my gym who was a type two diabetic. A few months after starting to work out, she went for a checkup and her doctor couldn't believe the results. 'Oh my God, what happened?' he said to her. 'Your levels are great.' The next time she came in, she told me that he'd taken her off the pills he'd been prescribing, and I started crying I was so happy. I love helping people, I love giving them the kind of hope people gave me. I want them to know that if I can do it, so can they."

But her passion for giving back didn't stop there. She started a Facebook Live program called *Thriving and Hope with Juanita*.

"Because I didn't want my outreach to be limited to only those who came into my gym. I wanted to help others, so they'd know there's hope for them too. That they can beat this, enjoy life, and live a long time. I wasn't sure how to do it at first, but I knew it had to be more than just some local cable access channel. One of my Christian sisters told me, 'God wants you to do this. He'll tell you when. You'll know.' I had done some Facebook videos to help sell the jewelry I make myself, and I realized that was it: live interviews on Facebook, and I made the cancer survivor who gave me the idea my first guest ever on the show. It's all about sharing your story, giving other people hope.

"And I have on anyone who wants to share their story. I leave posts that if they want to come on the show, just let me know. What I want to do is share as many stories as I can, all these amazing stories of survival people have to tell that can touch other people. Maybe someone in the audience will be able to relate because they're going through something similar. Maybe it's someone who's lost faith, and the show will help them build their faith back up. Give them hope and inspire them in some way so they can get back to the lives that they lost. I get so many messages because there are so many people out there who don't know how many others there are just like them, but they're out there. When I share my own story, I cry because of how far I've come. I cry because I'll never forget that pain and sadness when I first told my kids I had lung cancer. That was more than five years ago now. That's why I fought so hard, for them—my kids. Sometimes you have to overcome whatever life throws at you."

Juanita has since also gotten heavily involved with the LUNGevity Foundation and their Inhale for Life program.

"They asked me to do this video, and I was so honored to be part of a change when it comes to lung cancer treatment. I went to my first HOPE Summit in 2015 and met so many people who'd made it past the years they'd been given. At that point I'd only been given eighteen months to live, but their stories gave me hope and made me realize that I didn't need to let that timetable define me. I even did a boot camp there, because I wanted other survivors to see what they were capable of. I kicked their butts, and they loved every minute of it because it made them feel so alive. These women couldn't believe it, and I thought to myself, *Hey, I'm doing something. I'm giving back! I'm helping other lung cancer survivors.* And they couldn't have been more grateful."

Juanita has also played the role of a lung cancer patient advocate for Pfizer, serving on the pharmaceutical company's steering committee, and she was right there when Pfizer launched an exciting new drug. But it's her work with current patients she enjoys the most.

"If I can give them just a spark of hope, the size of a mustard seed… For as long as I'm on this earth, I'm going to do everything I possibly can. And when I meet a patient I can help, I know it's because God brought them to me."

But like all the survivors you've met in this book, Juanita has had her share of dark moments as well.

"The worst was after my second traditional chemo treatment," she recalls. "I remember feeling so sick. I remember how much I wanted to live, but I was so sick I didn't think I was going to. I couldn't eat, could barely drink—that was my lowest moment. My husband was yelling at me to eat because the doctors told me I needed to get my strength back—even someone who loved me was angry and disappointed. So when I was alone, I looked up at the ceiling and said, 'Lord, I can't do this. If this is my time go, just take me and take care of my kids. Guide them, protect them, and don't let them go through what I'm going through.' I couldn't do the chemo anymore and all I wanted was a protein shake, but the hospital staff wouldn't make one for me. So my husband stood up for me and insisted and, sure enough, they made me one. It tasted so good, I asked him to get me another and I drank that one too. Then that night I woke up to find my son, a freshman in college, sleeping in the bed next to me. When I saw him there, something snapped in me and I knew I had to live. I remember looking up at the ceiling. 'I have to live. I take it all back, Lord,' I said out loud. 'I have to live for my kids. Help me live for them.' Seeing my son sleeping in bed next to me ignited a spark in me."

I love the image of Juanita squeezing everything possible out of a workout with the same grit and determination she's used to beat cancer. She's a metaphor for so many out there who refuse to quit fighting, a poster child for the strength it takes to beat the odds and render lung cancer a part of a patient's life instead of allowing life to be defined by it. Indeed, Juanita chooses to define her life as a continuous series of repetitions strung together in spite of her disease instead of because of it. But she also talks about how cancer has made her a better person.

"It made me stronger, stronger in my faith. It made me grateful for the small things in life, whereas before I was living in the world without really knowing how I should be living. And it made me humble. The things I used to take for granted I don't take for granted anymore. I think I was a negative person before. Now I'm not, now I'm very positive. I can even see a cure for cancer. If they could do it with polio and smallpox, they can do it with cancer."

My mind flashes back to that initial image from the video of Juanita dead-lifting more than my body weight, the exertion squeezed tautly over her expression in a manner that makes failure an impossibility.

"My pastor tells me that I want to save the world, at least every lung cancer patient, and he's right. 'I don't know if God's going to give you the gift of healing,' he tells me, 'but He's given you a different one. You may not realize it, but you're using it every single day. Maybe not exactly the way you want to as much as the way God wants you to.' And I believe He'll bring other opportunities my way so I can continue doing what I'm doing.

"I'm just getting started."

I thought you might like to learn a bit about some recent initiatives undertaken by the GO2 Foundation following the merger of the Bonnie J. Addario Lung Cancer Foundation with the Lung Cancer Alliance. The merger allows initiatives like this to gain even more traction and efficacy. They are presented here in the form of posts that appeared on our website in June of 2020.

VA AND GO2 FOUNDATION PARTNER TO IMPROVE OUTCOMES FOR VETERANS AT RISK OF LUNG CANCER

A historic milestone was reached today with the exciting announcement that the Department of Veterans Affairs (VA) and GO2 Foundation for Lung Cancer (GO2 Foundation) have established a formal partnership to advance lifesaving screening and care for our military men and women at greater risk for lung cancer. One of GO2 Foundation's core priorities is educating people at risk for lung cancer and facilitating access to early detection screenings and care that can save lives. Working to better support Veterans who are at elevated risk and incidence for lung cancer than the civilian population has been a key focus of our organization for years.

This partnership allows GO2 Foundation to offer the VA educational and technical assistance and to collaborate on ways to improve Veterans' access to high-quality screening and care in communities where they live. This partnership will strengthen and accelerate efforts to change the reality of lung cancer for our service members. It will help break down barriers to save lives.

The announcement could not come at a better time as lung cancer advocates are gathering virtually at the 2020 Lung Cancer Voices Summit to call on Congress to increase funding for lung cancer research. As more breakthroughs are achieved, the VA-GO2 Foundation partnership picks up the baton and carries it forward to Veterans who will benefit from these lifesaving endeavors.

LUNG CANCER REGISTRY LAUNCHES LANDMARK SURVEY ON WOMEN'S SEXUAL HEALTH

The Lung Cancer Registry has launched a landmark new survey on the impact of lung treatments on women's sexual health. The aim is to explore the magnitude of the problem and give researchers and clinicians new insights to improve the quality of life for women lung cancer survivors.

Sexual Health Assessment in Women with Lung Cancer (SHAWL) is the first comprehensive look at the impact of a lung cancer diagnosis on a woman's sexual quality of life. The SHAWL survey asks intimate and blunt questions about women's sexual activity, questions that don't get asked enough according to the lead investigator.

"We're working hard to keep lung cancer patients alive longer, but no one stopped to ask these women questions about their sexual health," said Narjust Duma, MD, assistant professor at the University of Wisconsin School of Medicine and Public Health and SHAWL's principal investigator. "Sexual Health Assessment in Women with Lung Cancer is designed to pull back the curtain, collect the data, and help researchers study these too often unspoken side effects."

"We hope that SHAWL empowers women to share their stories, not just with the Lung Cancer Registry but also with their doctors," said Laurie Fenton Ambrose, Co-Founder, President & CEO, GO2 Foundation for Lung Cancer. "There's a huge gap in our understanding of the impact of therapies on women's sexual dysfunction. GO2 Foundation for Lung Cancer is excited to be able to help researchers tackle this important issue."

All people diagnosed with lung cancer or their caregivers are invited to take part in the Lung Cancer Registry. Women patients who sign up for the Lung Cancer Registry will be asked to complete the SHAWL survey.

About the Lung Cancer Registry

The Lung Cancer Registry is a community for people with all forms of lung cancer. Powered by data from patients and caregivers, this platform gives those most affected by lung cancer a voice. Registered patients, caregivers, clinicians, and researchers can access the de-identified information.

Founded in 2016, the Lung Cancer Registry is a core program of the GO2 Foundation for Lung Cancer. The Registry joined forces with the American Lung Association and the International Association for the Study of Lung Cancer to expand the effort to advance research for the world's deadliest cancer.

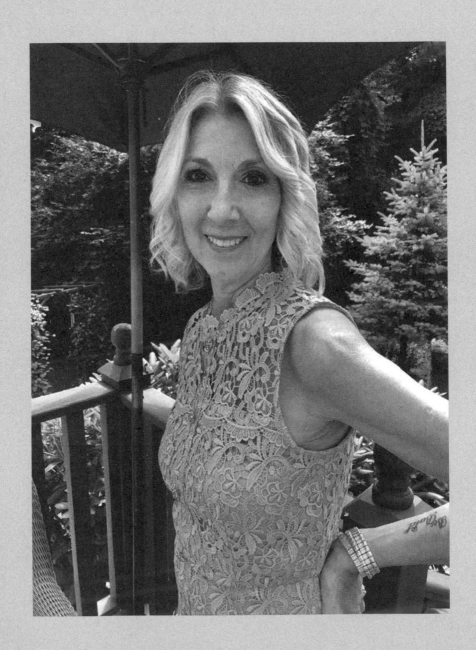

15

Lois Iannone

"I never had any symptoms, not a single warning sign," reflects Lois Iannone on her diagnosis of stage IV lung cancer between Thanksgiving and Christmas in 2018. "I was obsessed with staying healthy, so involved with preventative medicine. I couldn't even remember a time I was sick. I didn't even get colds."

That is, until she and her husband, Julio, a tailor who's a longtime local fixture on the East Side of Providence, Rhode Island, were visiting their daughter in Florida over the Thanksgiving holiday.

"I had a little sore throat and what felt like a bad chest cold, that feeling of congestion just below the neck. I didn't really feel sick, I wasn't blowing my nose, so I picked up some Mucinex, figuring that might help. I cooked the turkey and we had a wonderful day. But I know my body, and something just didn't feel right. I called my primary as soon as I got home, and she told me to come right in because she knows I'm never sick. She checked me out, and every time she asked me to take a breath in, I'd cough. So she prescribed two antibiotics, gave me a nebulizer treatment and an inhaler. I asked her if I should get a chest X-ray to check for pneumonia, and my doctor said why not? When I got home, the phone was ringing. My doctor had just read the X-ray."

"'It doesn't look good,' she said."

"So I asked her what that meant."

"'You need a CT scan. I've scheduled you for Friday—tomorrow.'"

"She called me the next day after my scan, when I was in the car driving home from running some errands, with the results."

"'Lois, this looks like lung cancer.'"

"So that's how I got diagnosed. That's the moment that changed my life forever."

A mutual friend who'd heard of Lois's plight and knew of my work recommended she reach out to me. We scheduled a phone call and spoke for well over an hour, covering all the bases we could initially. Unlike a lot of recently diagnosed lung cancer patients, Lois could not look back and see any indication or potential symptom of the disease going back years or months. A dedicated yoga practitioner who'd just accumulated the five hundred hours required to become a certified instructor, she was also still a practicing lawyer specializing in family law. She had been a light smoker decades earlier, long before she reached her mid-sixties, but that was before the yoga, the organic diet, the swearing off of sugar and soda. In other words, Lois was living a prototypical "clean" life, doing all the things you're supposed to do with regard to food, exercise, and preventative checkups. All things considered, and with no family history of cancer, she seemed a prime candidate to live to be a hundred.

"I went from that," she tells me, "to being told that if I didn't start chemo immediately, I might not last another week, maybe not even until the weekend. They told me my left atrium had collapsed. They tapped my lungs and pulled out a half gallon of fluid. The good news was a second CT scan and MRI showed the cancer hadn't spread. The bad news was my initial scan showed tumors everywhere through my lungs, and I mean everywhere. My chest scans were full of these white dots."

We speak on the phone as we did in our initial call in which she sounded like so many other recently diagnosed patients I speak with. In that call, Lois related how having a port installed to facilitate her chemotherapy infusions proved to be a tortuous procedure, and then, the week after receiving her first chemo treatment, she and Julio made the one-hour drive from Providence to Boston's Dana-Farber Cancer Institute, one of the finest anywhere, for a second opinion.

"First off," the doctor told them, "if you didn't have that chemotherapy treatment, you wouldn't have lived long enough to get here."

"So how long do I have?" Lois asked him, not mincing words.

The doctor looked up from the scans he'd been reviewing. "Four to six weeks," he said bluntly.

Lois and Julio cried all the way home. They held hands the whole time, hers trembling in his grasp.

"I was never going to never see my grandchildren grow up. My husband and I worked our whole lives for retirement and now there would be no retirement. My world was crumbling, and I had no control and no avenue to give me answers or explanations. It was the lowest point of my life, my darkest moment ever. In that moment, I had no hope at all."

The doctor at Dana-Farber had also told them that the treatment plan prescribed by Rhode Island's Roger Williams Medical Center was identical to what they would do. There was, thus, no real reason to travel to Boston, and Lois committed to the full six-treatment chemotherapy protocol that was supplemented with a cutting-edge immunotherapy drug that works with a patient's own immune system to help them fight certain cancers. The good news was that her type of lung cancer, non-small cell, made Lois a great fit for the drug that had shown extremely promising results in stage IV patients, especially in combination with chemotherapy. The bad news still hanging over her was the diagnosis from Dana-Farber that she likely had only a month left to live regardless, six weeks at the most.

But Lois remembers the exact moment she had a feeling she was turning a corner, right around the end of that six-week window the Dana-Farber oncologist had predicted in giving her a death sentence.

"They'd just started me on this targeted therapy, and as the infusion hit its peak, I started feeling this burning right at the site where the cancer was in my lungs. It felt like the drug was, literally, melting the tumors."

And sure enough, an initial follow-up CT scan prior to her third treatment showed significant improvement at around the twelve-week mark, meaning Lois had already doubled the life span one of the finest cancer centers anywhere had given her, based solely on her scans. And that's the point: patients are far more than the sum total of their scans. Scans don't take attitude into account or the overall health of the patient in general. In Lois's case, her health was otherwise excellent, exemplary for a woman in her mid-sixties. She was, after all, a yoga instructor, which in and of itself didn't help much when at one point she was in bed for thirteen consecutive days. I ask Lois how she thinks she was able to defy the odds, getting a scan that was remarkably, if not miraculously, clear after she completed her sixth and final chemotherapy treatment.

"I learned to live in the now, not think about how I got here or where I was going. There's only today; the next minute, the next hour. I learned to live for today and worry about tomorrow when it gets here."

The very week I spoke with Lois, Merck, the targeted therapy's manufacturer, announced five-year data that showed "patients increased overall survival by 5X fold, to 23.2% in advanced lung cancer patients." Another set of results showed that "[This targeted therapy]— in combination with [another] drug to treat patients with metastatic nonsquamous NSCLC (Non-Small Cell Lung Cancer)—reduced the risk of death by 44%."

How impressive is that exactly? Before that targeted therapy came along, the five-year survival rate for patients with advanced lung cancer was only 5 percent in the United States.

Dr. Alice Shaw, a Massachusetts General Hospital lung cancer expert, told *Business Insider*, "This is really a pivotal study… A new standard of care."

"It's a very significant improvement," Dr. Roy Baynes, Merck's chief medical officer, added. "This really is a fundamental change in outcome for patients."

There's more. Dr. Baynes spoke to *Business Insider* about "identifying patients who might respond well to [targeted therapies] by using precision medicine techniques like genetic testing. In the longer term, [targeted therapy] also has big potential to be used earlier in the course of treating a patient's cancer."

So another "next big thing" on the horizon is using targeted therapy drugs after surgery to reduce the chances of reoccurrence and to extend remissions.

"While important progress has been made and recent therapeutic advances across a number of novel pathways have changed the paradigm for many patients, cancer remains a formidable foe," Dr. Baynes wrote recently on Merck's website. "The key to transforming the treatment of cancer is to continuously pursue discovery and clinical research that will allow us to help as many patients as possible. With that in focus, Merck is advancing a broad oncology development program that is exploring over 20 different novel mechanisms. This includes research designed to better understand how to deploy our medicines to the greatest effect and identifying those patients likely to benefit most. We know that cancer doesn't have a single cause or progress along a single pathway, so we will likely need to attack it in multiple ways. Advancing this goal requires drive and resilience to build and expand upon what has been achieved to date with a focus on improving the lives of patients. We have established a strong foundation and are excited to be leading the charge into the future."

An article in *Investor's Business Daily* from February of 2017 concurs.

"What if your body's immune system fought off deadly cancer cells just like it protects you from germs you encounter every day?" wrote

Allison Gatlin. "That's the goal of an emerging class of treatments called immuno-oncology, or I-O, drugs. 'Cancer cells are constantly occurring in everyone,' Tim Reilly, development lead for Bristol-Myers's early I-O pipeline, says. 'Every time we get out in the sunlight and get some UV exposure, there's a mutation to a cell that is technically now a mutated cell and is, technically, cancer. But our body eradicates that cell.' That's what a healthy immune system does. But, in some cases, aberrant cells evolve to outpace or outsmart the system, throwing off the body's natural homeostasis. Those cells then grow, becoming a cancerous tumor."

Drugs like the targeted therapy she was taking can change all that, all of which is music to Lois Iannone's ears. She plans to change her law practice to limited scope representation to continue helping people, while avoiding the stress so prevalent in family law. Indeed, empathy with her clients brought on such great stress, Lois is convinced it was one of the contributing factors to her getting sick. As for continuing to get better...

"Laughter is the best medicine. Laughter heals, that and getting plenty of sleep and physical activity. Yoga is meditation in motion. You're in the present moment, nowhere else. Now is beautiful. I love the now. The only thing on your mind is getting into a pose and holding it. This alone brings you mindfulness."

Lois especially enjoys teaching yoga to other cancer survivors at her daughter's studio in Jupiter, Florida. Hot yoga is too strenuous and draining right now, but she's happy to settle for the smooth and supple motions of the traditional brand, allowing her to go at her own pace, a student in the class instead of an instructor.

"When you get diagnosed with stage IV lung cancer, your mind goes to an entirely different place. I didn't know in that moment if I'd ever be able to exercise again. I wasn't thinking about it. All my energy was focused on staying alive, getting through this. But when your focus turns to getting better, you want to find the thing that makes you happy, gives you joy. You need to find joy once a day in something, no matter what, or how small, that is."

The challenge for lung cancer patients is *getting* to the now.

"The not knowing," Lois says, "the unknown, is horrible. It's like you don't even know what's going to happen in the next hour. I just wanted to be aware of what was coming next. The disease is in control, and nothing and no one can change that. I had an incredible support system, but I was the only one who knew exactly what I was going through physically. You're with yourself. You're with your thoughts. You're in this little tornado and there's no room inside for anyone else.

"And you get angry. Why me? What did I do to deserve this? I mean, what the hell, why do I have to go through all this. Other people go to Burger King and eat french fries and I'm the one going through this? I got angrier at the beginning, especially the day before chemo. I don't get angry as much now because I'm feeling better. But I look at anger as a kind of coping mechanism."

Lois is quick to point out that there are some positive things as well that emerged during her chemotherapy treatments.

"Our family grew a lot closer. I find myself grateful for everything, and I've stopped taking things, even the simplest things, for granted. You're happier because you appreciate everything so much more, especially people. Cancer doesn't just test you; it brings out the best in you and in the people around you. I feel stronger than the day I got sick. Everything I'm doing, I'm doing for myself."

I ask Lois what advice she'd give a recently diagnosed lung cancer patient.

"First of all, write everything down. I have a folder at home with medical reports, scans, along with all the questions I've asked and answers I've gotten. Second, don't lose hope. Never lose hope. Third, enjoy the now. Fourth, laugh until your belly can't take it anymore. And, fifth, call you, Bonnie, just like I did, and we talked for over an hour in that initial phone call. You wanted to know more about me, you wanted to see my medical records. You were the first person I could really talk to about this, because you'd been through it too. I think you were validating me and my feelings, and you sent me that handbook."

The handbook Lois is referring to is called *Navigating Lung Cancer: 360 Degrees of Hope*. I'm listed as the author and that's me on the cover, but the book is really a compilation of knowledge from experts about what a recently diagnosed lung cancer patient should do, step by step. The GO2 Foundation makes it available for free, for any patient who requests a copy.

"It contained so much invaluable information," Lois continues. "I wish I'd had it from day one because I would have known the questions to ask, what to expect, what I'd be facing next. I kept asking you, 'What does this mean?' I needed to know so I could better understand my cancer. And I cried as soon as I got off the phone call with you, because I felt good for the first time since my diagnosis. The best antidote to lung cancer is information, because there are people out there who know what you don't."

More than a year has passed since our initial interview, and in our most recent call Lois told me that her prognosis has become so positive her doctors are strongly considering taking her off the Keytruda. She will not only be medication-free at that point but also cancer-free.

And what about Lois's three wishes for the future?

"Find a cure for lung cancer, all cancers," she says. "To live a full, vibrant life and not be sick, not be homebound, not have to rely on other people. And I'm happy now, as happy as I've ever been, and I want to see other people be happy."

BIOMARKER TESTING

Biomarker testing (also called molecular testing) looks for biological changes in genes or proteins, like EGFR or ALK, that may be associated with your cancer. In most cases, this involves testing a piece of tissue from the cancer (a biopsy).

Get Tested Now

GO2 Foundation for Lung Cancer has a partnership with a leading precision medicine company, Perthera, to offer biomarker testing to patients. To get started, call us at 1-800-298-2436 or email support@ go2foundation.org to request a call about biomarker testing. Our HelpLine team will connect you with a Treatment and Trial Navigator from LungMATCH, who will explain how the program works. Personalized treatment recommendations will be provided for you to discuss with your doctor. Get started today!

Who Should Be Tested?

Due to the exploding number of treatment options, *we recommend all patients with non-small cell lung cancer be tested*. We also offer biomarker testing to those with other types of lung cancer. For additional information, contact our LungMATCH specialist at 1-800-298-2436 or support@go2foundation.org. Download our biomarker testing flyer for an easy overview.

Why Is it Important?

Because every person's cancer is different. This testing offers you and your treatment team the information you need to identify the best treatment for your individual case.

Treatment Options

Many of the changes that have been identified in genes and proteins of those with lung cancer occur in a small percentage of those impacted by the disease. There are only approved treatments for some of those changes. If there is not an approved treatment for the changes in your cancer, there may be a clinical trial that would be a good match for you.

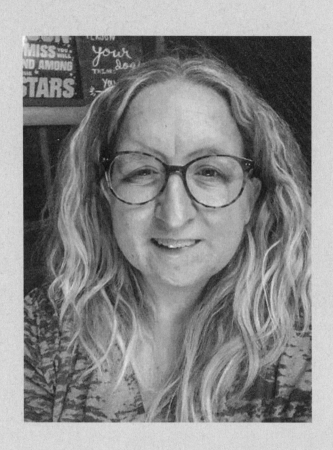

16

Diane Spry

One of the highlights of Diane Spry's winter of 2019 was venturing to Soldier Field on a frigid January day to watch her beloved Chicago Bears play the Philadelphia Eagles in an NFL playoff game. Along with other survivors, she was the guest of Chris Draft, a former NFL player who's started a foundation to support lung cancer.

"We met for the first time at a HOPE Summit," Diane tells me, referring to a survivorship conference sponsored by LUNGevity. "Chris is a huge advocate for lung cancer, and he gets tickets for survivors and makes sure they're recognized, to draw attention to the disease."

With good reason. Chris Draft, you see, lost his own wife, LaKeasha, to lung cancer in December of 2011. A healthy thirty-eight-year-old woman and professional dancer, she never smoked a day in her life. Her diagnosis came just a year before her death and, like many, it came out of nowhere.

"Right now," Chris told *Essence* magazine in February 2012, "with Team Draft our goal is to change the face of lung cancer. We want people to see that anybody can get lung cancer, and the cure for it is just as critical as breast cancer, or any cancer. We've got to find a way to identify it earlier. Keasha was this strong, healthy woman, who was all of a sudden short of breath. Had she caught it during stage three, instead of four, it could have really increased her chances of survival. We're going to celebrate her life and the type of person she was and we want others to grab hold of her spirit and make a difference. There's no clear answer in terms of what can be done to identify it early enough. Keasha didn't smoke, she was a dancer, she was fit, and she was healthy. That's why people need to see faces like hers and continue to be inspired. We want to build an excitement about making a difference. I want to put a picture of Keasha right in front of researchers' faces, so when the doctors and scientists are doing their research, they see her right there smiling, and it can hopefully give them that little extra push. If we could push things ahead, and give someone else another week, it makes a huge difference. Team Draft was launched at our wedding. She wanted to fight. She wanted to stand up. Continuing this allows her to do that."

Reading those words, I can't help but be struck that the drugs that saved Diane Spry's life weren't around in 2012 when LaKeasha Draft was diagnosed. Diane was diagnosed in 2014 and calls the people she's met as a result the silver lining in the cloud of lung cancer. In fact, she has a survivors' support group in Chicago that call themselves the Silver Lining Sisters.

"We've formed a real community that's defined by the fact that we're all fighting the same battle. We all understand what everyone is going through, and we're there for each other when one of us finally loses the battle. When I went to that football game, it made me think that we have our own little cheerleading group. When I have scans, they have scans, and the whole process, dealing with the disease, is made so much easier by knowing you have people in your corner."

Diane speaks of meeting a young, recently diagnosed Filipina woman online and building a long-distance relationship with her through social media. Then they actually met in person in Washington, DC, at the LUNGevity International Conference on Lung Cancer, formerly the HOPE Summit. They may have changed the name of the conference, but they haven't taken hope out of it or the lives of Diane and the other Silver Lining Sisters.

"Most of the time, when you meet someone online, there's no realness to it. They're just a screen name, that's all. It's different when that someone is a fellow lung cancer patient. That makes things so much more real because we can relate to each other and understand what we're each going through. A common bond."

Diane's portal into the world of lung cancer advocacy was LUNGevity, but she's also attended events sponsored by the Bonnie Addario Lung Cancer Foundation and will continue to do so under our new auspices at the GO2 Foundation.

"That's the thing about all these lung cancer organizations. They're not run by hired guns or political appointees. They're run by fellow lung cancer survivors. There was a time where that wasn't the case because the survival for lung cancer patients was so grim. The change is testament to how much things have improved and are still improving. Used to be you got a diagnosis and would die in three months, a year at most. Now lung cancer survivors are living ten years or more, and that gives us the people to stand up and fight, stand up and say, 'Let's live five years, ten years, more. I'm still here. Let's do this.'"

Like her fellow Silver Lining Sisters, a group that includes Juanita Segura, whom you've already met, Diane is passionate about advocacy.

"I share my story because that kind of story was what I needed to hear when I was first diagnosed as a thirty-year-old nonsmoker. I needed to hear about more people my age, my demographic, who have gone through what I was going through. I share my story whenever I have the opportunity because there are people out there who need to hear it. I wear a LUNGevity T-shirt, and whenever anybody asks me about it, I'll talk their ear off for fifteen minutes in a line for a restaurant or something like that. I'll talk to anybody, because everybody needs to hear about my experience, what I have to say.

"For some people," Diane continues after a pause, "talking about the disease becomes like reliving their most painful experiences. There are people in our community who even take Facebook breaks, but I'm not one of them. I stick with it. I'm involved on a daily basis through these Facebook groups that I moderate. Having lung cancer has taught me the value of time, and I'm not going to waste any."

Diane's case highlights another issue that often follows a lung cancer diagnosis, that being the financial strains it places on the patient and their family. With the overriding emphasis placed on a patient getting their physical health back, short shrift is often given to the toll the treatment process also takes on financial well-being.

"At the time I was diagnosed," she recalls, "I was working full time, hanging out with my boyfriend, taking day trips on the weekends, and traveling. I had a routine. When I got sick, I lost my independence. I couldn't do the work I loved, or any work, for eight months, which meant I had no money coming in. I had to rely so heavily on my boyfriend. I had to move in with my sister, where I'm still living today. So cancer didn't just steal my health, it stole my life. I thought about a lot of things when I was first diagnosed, but I didn't think about the economic toll that lung cancer takes. I was only able to work part time until very recently and stayed afloat only because I had people to lean on. My sister paid a lot of my bills. Friends held a benefit in my honor to help pay for the day-to-day costs of lung cancer, like traveling back and forth to Boston for a year when I was enrolled in a clinical trial at Dana-Farber."

This isn't something a lot of people or patients are comfortable talking about, and the financial strain Diane is alluding to often affects caregivers as much as patients, on top of the emotional strain. Think about the stress of worrying about how the bills are going to get paid on top of the challenge of fighting a disease like lung cancer. It takes all your energy and passion to beat it, leaving nothing left in the tank to cope with the economic burdens that pile on as well. Diane's friends and family, though, rallied to her side, and her boyfriend was there for her every minute of every day.

Fortunately, Diane's situation had been eased substantially by the University of Chicago, where she's being treated, paying for the bulk of her medical care, which leaves her better equipped to focus on the day-to-day bills and expenses now that she is five years into her treatment.

"I'm trying to get my life back—that's where my focus is. I'm still working part time and picked up a second part-time job. With my new expanded schedule, I have to worry about things such as packing a lunch. I have to coordinate when I will do tasks such as going to the bank or post office. And I'm looking for a full-time position. My boyfriend and I got married. We're still living with my sister until we find a house to buy for ourselves, and we're looking. With my increased hours at work, I have also seen a bit more in the old paycheck, which is always nice. I'm able to go shopping for what I need and not have to depend on my family and friends for a change. I'm on the right track."

Diane is focused on looking ahead. She can't get back the time or toll lung cancer took on her—no lung cancer patient can. But she looks ahead toward a future highlighted by new and even more effective drugs entering the market to fight the disease.

"I was on a drug originally prescribed for thyroid cancer for two years. It was pretty toxic and had a lot of side effects, but it helped keep me alive."

Diane is off that drug now and receiving a new targeted therapy that has restored her quality of life while keeping her lung cancer at bay.

That same targeted therapy is being studied for its effectiveness in treating colon, breast, pancreatic, stomach, and other cancers, in addition to melanoma. Turnabout being fair play, there are numerous other cancer drugs out there that may someday similarly work wonders for lung cancer patients, in addition to the next wave of therapies developed toward that specific end. The cancer world, you might say, is determined to share the wealth, and that's a great thing for all cancer sufferers.

Even more determined to do her part toward that end, Diane has recently taken over the coordination of Breathe Deep Kankakee, a 5K walk/run to raise money for lung cancer.

"This is how I can help fight this disease. And since the event takes place right where I live, it gives the opportunity to bring the fight home to my own neighborhood. I want people to realize that what happened to me can happen to them, their friends, their family, their neighbors. For me, this run is about bringing lung cancer advocacy home. We started small with only fifty-seven participants, but that's fifty-seven new soldiers out there battling lung cancer."

Based on her own experiences, I ask Diane her advice for newly diagnosed lung cancer patients.

"That's always been a really difficult question for me, because there's no pat answer. Normally, I listen to their story, starting with where they are with their staging, diagnosis, and biomarkers. What I say, my response, is based on what they tell me. But the part of my experience I share with them across the board is the part I just shared with a coworker recently diagnosed with stage IV lung cancer: 'I'm still here after five years,' I told him. 'And you can be too.' That was a huge thing for him to hear, for any lung cancer patient to hear."

We heard from Dr. Pasi Jänne, director of the Lowe Center for Thoracic Oncology at Dana-Farber Cancer Institute in Boston, just prior to chapter 3. Here's Part Two of his thoughts on the state of lung cancer treatment today.

The reason I come to work every day is very clear: there are people who need help, who have lung cancer and need better therapies to treat their disease. Everything we do is about making those people better. And we've had some pronounced successes that fuel the process further. Because if something good can happen to one subset of patients, then it can happen for others. It's all about coming to better understand the disease in order to improve outcomes.

Sometimes we lose patients. We just ran out of therapies for them, and it hurts. It's always a disappointment when that happens, but it motivates and inspires us to want to do more so that someday we never run out of treatments to keep people alive. Those day-to-day frustrations are unavoidable. But what's not avoidable is seeing people who've missed opportunities because certain therapies weren't offered them. I see patients all the time who could have benefited from something but never got the chance.

We've gotten to the point where the first thing we want to know post-diagnosis is what type of lung cancer it is specifically as defined by the genetic subset of the disease. And the second thing we want to know is whether we have an existing therapy that particular patient's cancer will more likely respond to. The specifics of the cancer dictate the specifics of the treatment.

Discovering the EGFR genetic mutation back in 2004, for example, helped us understand that there are individual patients who can benefit from targeted therapies. Cancers can outsmart drugs; they can keep growing in spite of the presence of those drugs and ongoing treatment. The cancers mutate, and these new mutations prevent the drug from binding to those cells. Can we find why that's the case? Is there something that could make the drug outsmart the cancer instead of the reverse happening? It's a chemistry angle more than a biological one. Since the EGFR mutation shows up in so many lung cancer patients, my team worked with chemists to develop treatment entities that could inhibit EGFR in ways never thought possible. I published a paper in 2009 that for the first time described EGFR inhibitors that could potentially prevent the mutations, which helped open up a brand-new area to clinical research. And I was able to do that because of my expertise in dual disciplines that are seldom practiced together.

See, a lot of chemists are more interested in discovering the next element on the periodic table than treating cancer, so employing chemistry this way is a relatively new thing. Nobody can achieve such things on their own, working in their own thought bubble. You have to talk to each other. You have to interact with these other disciplines to fully and effectively treat patients with therapies that maximize their survivability. You need to look at the problem from various perspectives to come up with the kind of novel insights that are much more difficult to achieve than for a single discipline working alone. I see that happening more and more, thanks in large part to academia's interest in this particular field and this particular disease. You can do things in academics you just can't do in business.

So my overall message is one of hope. It's about staying ahead of the game, thinking about and waiting for the next big thing that may emerge. More and more lung cancer patients are alive five, even ten years later. I can see us shifting more to a place where lung cancer is more of a chronic but manageable disease, as opposed to feeling like an immediate death sentence. We may not be able to cure the disease, but our patients will be able to live far longer with their cancers. It used to be, when I started out in the 1990s, that holidays were an especially difficult time for lung cancer patients because patients wondered if this was going to be the last one. That doesn't even enter our thinking anymore.

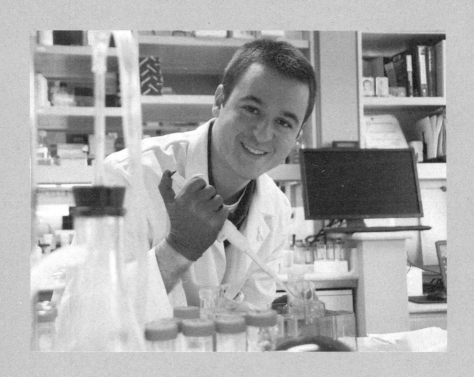

17

Matt Hiznay

Matt Hiznay has a remarkable memory, not that he'd necessarily need one to remember the day he was diagnosed with stage IV lung cancer.

"I was thinking, 'I'm twenty-four, I'm a lifelong nonsmoker…I'm not supposed to get cancer.'"

That was over nine years ago, August of 2011 to be exact, right about the time Matt was entering his second year of medical school. A cruel irony, but one that did nothing to cushion the shock. Nor did he ever suspect the lingering dry cough that finally sent him to his primary care doctor was lung cancer, not in his wildest nightmares.

"I remember that cough, but cancer was the last thing in my head. I blamed allergies and the fact that I was living in a new city with new things to be allergic to. I figured it was just something in the air."

Which, of course, it wasn't.

"I'd studied science as a college undergrad, and being a medical student at the time, I knew the cancer was growing and dividing every moment we weren't treating it. I wanted to know exactly what it was

231

so we could throw the kitchen sink at it. I was young and physically fit, so I felt good about my chances. Getting sick at twenty-four meant my body would be able to handle a lot more than even slightly older patients. The immediate thought for me wasn't that I'm going to die; I was thinking instead of what might be the best possible place to get treated. But then my mind started playing games with me about the treatment not working and this being my final chapter. There was no family history of cancer on either side, so it wasn't like there was a family member who knew all the dos and don'ts. When you're young, it's easy to think you're invincible, and it's amazing how quickly you learn that you're mortal."

A week later, on August 17, 2011, to be exact, Matt traveled from his native Youngstown, Ohio, to the prestigious Cleveland Clinic to meet with his oncologist.

"We talked about potential plans and protocols. I checked some boxes for genetic testing, so that was good. But some of those boxes raised flags for him. He said he was going to send the tumor out to be tested, but I wanted to start traditional chemo right away on the assumption I might not have the markers. Good thing the doctor agreed with me too, because by September 1 the cancer had spiraled out of control and I ended up in the ICU. If I hadn't pushed for the chemo, I would have died at my parents' house before I even got the genetic testing results."

I hear time and time again about the importance of not only early diagnosis but early treatment. Lung cancer is extremely virulent and moves through the body like wildfire. It has the potential to be like the killer cyborg in the first *Terminator* movie, about which the human sent back in time to protect the cyborg's target says, "It can't be bargained with, it can't be reasoned with. It doesn't feel pity, or remorse, or fear. And it absolutely will not stop, ever, until you are dead." In the end, though, the cyborg fails in its ultimate mission. Its victim fights back and ultimately wins.

Just like Matt did, thanks to insisting on starting treatment a mere week after his diagnosis.

"Patient advocacy is beyond important. It's daunting to have a loved one get sick, and I was beyond fortunate that my wife, then only my girlfriend, and my mother were there for me. Even as a med student, I didn't know all the ins and outs of cancer. Sure, I can tell you a lot more now than I could then because, between the three of us, we were researching all the time. We all like to think of the oncologist and their team as being superhuman and all-knowing, but things are happening so fast, it's hard for even them to keep up with everything. I wanted to know exactly what I was facing and how best to beat it. The bad news: it was an extremely aggressive form of the disease caused by a genetic mutation. The good news: it could be treated with a brand-new targeted therapy that the Food and Drug Administration had approved the same day I was diagnosed."

Matt and I meet up at the American Society of Clinical Oncology convention at McCormick Place in Chicago. It's a massive convention center, but we're both staying at the Renaissance Blackstone Chicago, which is on-site, so we're able to snare a table at a posh lobby lounge called Timothy's Hutch. It's busy, the rattle of glasses and composite of voices forming background noise that quickly gets drowned out when we start talking. Matt looks healthy and fit, nothing to even suggest his eight-year battle with lung cancer. His eyes flash with hope, seeming to see past me toward whatever future now awaits him thanks to the innovative therapies that have changed the face of treatment. He's a poster child for both this insidious scourge affecting more and more young people as well as the leaps and bounds medicine has made that have kept him alive.

"The Lord really does work in mysterious ways," Matt continues. "Looking back, I remember thinking I'd been dealt a terrible hand getting cancer and there was no way I was going to be in that five percent that had the ALK mutation that would have made me eligible for targeted therapies. I was rushed to the hospital on September 1 and stopped breathing on September 2. Then a week later I found out I had the ALK mutation, and a week after that I was on a targeted therapy."

His heart actually stopped multiple times, due to all the fluid around his heart and lungs.

"That targeted therapy saved my life. By November of 2011, I was in remission. Then in May, I noticed some swelling in my left shoulder, and in the deepest, darkest part of my mind I knew what it was."

The cancer was indeed back, and Matt's Cleveland Clinic oncologist, Dr. Nathan Pennell, got him into a clinical trial that worked well enough to shrink the tumor, but standard chemotherapy was needed to destroy it. And when the cancer returned yet again, Matt was treated with radiation. In March 2015, the cancer came back for a fourth time and he enrolled in yet another clinical trial, this time a Phase I trial, which meant little to nothing was known about the drug's side effects and potential toxicity levels.

"I wasn't scared," Matt said in "Alive—and Thriving—Thanks to Cancer Research," a post for the Cleveland Clinic website. "There's not much that can scare me anymore. I have a lot of faith in these types of drugs and therapies, and I've been fortunate that I've responded. Enrolling in a clinical trial is one of the most altruistic things you can do—letting yourself be studied and scrutinized at an extremely high scientific level to help the patients of tomorrow."

In Matt's case, the drug in question also helped a patient of today: him. And he's been on it, successfully, ever since.

"People take their diabetes or heart disease pills, and I take my cancer pills. I've been on three different targeted therapies now, done traditional chemo and radiation, and I want to believe my cancer is now being successfully managed. I don't know if lung cancer will ever get to where heart disease is when it comes to managing, because cancer can be trickier. But I think we have a chance of achieving real success in making the disease controlled or chronic. 'Cure' is a great goal to shoot for, but 'chronic and controlled' is a much more likely outcome."

As that same post for the Cleveland Clinic notes, Matt has begun to pay it forward by furthering medical research himself. Instead of finishing medical school, he joined the Cleveland Clinic's molecular medicine PhD program and currently works in the lab of researcher Richard Padgett, who's studying how mutations in a step of gene processing drive cancer growth. On his first day, Matt encountered a fellow graduate student, Hannah (Stubbs) Picariello, who had worked on the clinical trial of the drug that triggered his first remission.

"Thank you for saving my life," he told her.

Our server sets fresh diet sodas before us on fresh napkins as well. She smiles warmly before taking her leave, as if she has some intuitive notion of what we're discussing.

"That woman I was talking about—Hannah—had just graduated and was out celebrating when she got word the drug had actually worked on patients. When I got sick, I was ready to start my second year of med school. I wanted to be a doctor, a healer. When I became a patient, quite naively I figured I'd survive this and all I'd have to do is take this pill for the rest of my life. I went back to Toledo to pick up where I left off, ready to sign a lease, when my cancer recurred for the first time. That's when I realized I was in for a lifelong battle. A lot of med school is physically demanding, and I didn't feel I could hold myself up to the bar I needed to. I made the difficult decision to leave med school but still wanted to be a healer, and I knew my way around a research lab because I'd worked in one over the summer I got sick. So I enrolled in graduate school and was lucky enough to land a research position at the very Cleveland Clinic where I was being treated myself, in a lab that studies leukemia."

On top of everything else, all the chemotherapy robbed Matt of the use of his left arm. While occupational therapy has restored a measure of function, it wouldn't have been nearly enough to practice medicine or even continue in medical school. So his decision to leave and pursue the medical profession along a different track proved fortuitous indeed.

"I'll admit my foresight only goes a half year into the future now," he tells me. "I don't even see a full year ahead. Everything was going along just as I'd planned it. The world was my oyster and nothing was going to get in my way. Then cancer came along."

I ask him if cancer stole his dreams, as it had for so many like the physician Paul Kalanithi, as so wondrously described in *When Breath Becomes Air* and in an earlier chapter featuring Paul's widow, Lucy.

"It made me come up with new dreams," Matt says. "I don't regret making the choices I made. My arm and hand recovered enough to allow me to type a one hundred-fifty-page dissertation for grad school. I enjoy reading and writing, and I've done a lot of speaking. In fact, I present findings to the doctors and nurses who are going to put them to use treating the very patients I can't."

He pauses, his mind moving in another direction.

"This time of year—May 11, 2011, near the end of my first year of medical school—was when my grandfather died. This is the time of year when memories I keep locked up the rest of the year under multiple locks and keys open up. I had to look up all the dates, the benchmarks. I had to ask my family to re-create everything for me because I was in a fog. I wanted to create a timeline for posterity."

I ask if he considers himself a miracle, given that such a small percentage of stage IV lung cancer patients live five years, particularly when diagnosed so young.

"I don't want to give myself the jinx," Matt says with a smile. "So I consider what's happened to me miraculous, but I don't consider myself to be a miracle. I thank God every night to be alive and ask what I'm supposed to do with the time I got back. Because there has to be a reason why that happened."

His now wife, Aleksandra, a pharmacist at the Cleveland Clinic's Avon Hospital, stuck with him every bit of the way.

"She's the only person who had a choice in all this. I told her that no one in my family would hold it against her or bear her any ill will if she wanted to break up. She used some expletive and told me to shut up. We got engaged a year later and were married in 2014."

Matt is also quick to credit his mother.

"She's an all-or-nothing woman, and she took it upon herself to dig into the latest and upcoming therapies and to learn as much as she possibly could about the most renowned physicians when it came to lung cancer. Pain can blind you, robbing you of the ability to see even to the next day. My mom and Alex became my eyes in that respect, helping to steer me forward. In fact, it was my mom who found you and the Addario Foundation, remember?"

I do indeed. The idea that someone so young and who had never smoked could be diagnosed with lung cancer was striking. My daughter Danielle flew out to Cleveland to make a video to further debunk the myths associated with lung cancer.

"I became the really young guy who got sick and was saved by targeted therapies," Matt recalls.

He never set out to be a poster child, but now he is one for all the right reasons.

The American Society of Clinical Oncology (ASCO) conference is a positive place to be right now because this is the conference where the latest targeted therapies are unveiled, along with the data to support them. Matt is here in Chicago at ASCO as a guest of Pfizer, the pharmaceutical giant responsible for two of the drugs that have kept him alive. It's a part of the Go Boldly campaign that seeks to draw attention to the incredible work being done and progress made by Big Pharma, in part by teaming patients with the physicians and clinicians who discovered the drugs that have given them a second choice of life. For Matt that was Dr. Bob Abraham.

"My father was a World War Two veteran," Abraham opens in a May 2016 video that paired Matt with him to help get word out about the great strides being made in fighting lung cancer. "He was a tough guy. At the age of seventy-five, he was diagnosed with non-small cell lung cancer, and I watched what the disease did to a very strong man that I looked up to. I'm directing an organization of over four hundred scientists charged with the task of production of new anticancer agents from idea all the way through proof-of-concept studies."

That introduction is followed by Matt telling the story of his own diagnosis, intercut with shots of the Pfizer team at work developing the kind of drugs that saved his life.

"It's absolutely amazing," Matt says in the video, "the work that goes into making a drug."

"Immunotherapy is the latest wave of cancer drug discovery," Bob Abraham picks up. "We have the ability to turn on the patient's immune system and actually have the patient's own cells kill cancer. We're just extremely excited about the possibility that for the first time in history, we can induce durable and maybe even curative responses. When we have patients come and visit and tell us the benefit they've derived from a drug, it's just incredibly motivational."

"Through this Herculean effort of the people at Pfizer, my cancer is in remission," Matt adds. "To meet people who've been there since the beginning, to shake their hand and look them in the eye and say thank you, it's hard to even put what that feels like into words."

But pictures in the video more than make up for that, showing Matt and Dr. Abraham together, worth not just a thousand words or even a million. It's tough to put a word count on saving a life.

"Years of research have gone into this," Matt continues in the video, "and it's given me years back now. Five years ago, my hometown was crying for me to live. Two years ago, I got married."

"This is the most important time I've seen in cancer drug discovery in the past thirty years," Dr. Abraham adds as they walk out the door of the clinical facility into the sunlight. "I think about all the patients who aren't benefitting from the current therapies. We still have a lot to do here."

"Thanks to the tireless work of biopharmaceutical researchers and scientists," Stephen J. Ubl, president and chief executive officer of PhRMA (Pharmaceutical Research and Manufacturers of America), said in announcing the Go Boldly campaign, "we have entered a new era of medicine that is transforming the way we prevent and treat disease. This campaign spotlights their perseverance and unwavering commitment to American patients for whom we all work. We will also be convening events with stakeholders all across the country to discuss ways we can work together to make our health care system more responsive to the needs of patients."

The point is that the pharmaceutical industry is a key player in finally winning the war on cancer that began when Richard Nixon was still president, standing on the front lines along with doctors, advocates, and the patients themselves. Winning that war isn't an either/or proposition, and the researchers who saved Matt's life are on the verge of discovering far more innovative therapies that promise to save far more lives. Companies like Pfizer are responsible for getting us where we are today, and the same companies are moving us further toward making lung cancer a manageable condition so young men like Matt get to live a full life and older patients make it to their full life expectancy.

"Through partnerships and collaborations with other health care leaders," Ubl adds, "we will work to advance commonsense solutions that foster the continued development of new medicines, enhance the private marketplace, and provide patients with access to the newest and most innovative treatments."

Since 2000, companies associated with PhRMA have dedicated more than half a trillion dollars to the search for new cancer treatments and cures. And, according to the US National Library of Medicine, "In this analysis of US Securities and Exchange Commission filings for ten cancer drugs, the median cost of developing a single cancer drug was $648 million."

That staggering cost is hardly lost on Matt, who is alive because of funds allocated for such research.

"Cancer gives you a whole different perspective on life. You live your life in dog years, everything exaggerated and hyper-focused because you realize how lucky you are to be here. The first thing I tell recently diagnosed lung cancer patients is that this doesn't have to be the end."

What about his three wishes for the future?

"First and foremost, I wish for continued good health. Second, I wish for more options for therapy to keep me in good health should the current drug I'm on fail. Oh, and number three, I wish for the Cleveland Browns to win the Super Bowl."

You're about to meet Jill Feldman. In a book of original stories, hers is one that truly stands out, thanks to a family history that threatens our very understanding of lung cancer's origins. Indeed, as we've covered in many of the preceding chapters, all you need to get lung cancer is... lungs. In this post for LUNGevity, published in November 2015, Jill addresses that stigma in frank, passionate fashion, just as she did in the post that preceded chapter 8.

LET'S KILL THE STIGMA AND SAVE LIVES

Posted November 19, 2015, by Jill Feldman

Whoever said, "Sticks and stones may break your bones, but names/words will never hurt you," has never had lung cancer and heard those three words—*Did you smoke* or have to say those three words—*I never smoked*.

Those three words are toxic and create a serious barrier to diagnosis, treatment, and acceptance in the community. Even worse, they have created a barrier that is holding the lung cancer community back; a perpetuated stigma within the community itself. It's there and it's significant.

The stigma in the general public is so strong that survivors who have never smoked are forced to immediately, and constantly, declare three words ("I never smoked") to avoid the three words ("Did you smoke?") that imply self-infliction. Facing a lung cancer diagnosis is already an uphill battle—energy should be focused on health and survival, not on being forced to declare "innocence" or plead "guilty"!

It sounds like a harsh analogy, and that's because it is a harsh reality. The pervasive stigma is, unconsciously, dividing our community into two teams (innocent and guilty) at a time when we desperately need to unite. But, it's not easy to unite when we use the stigma itself to try and eliminate the stigma. There will always be a stigma if we are defined by what kind of smoker we are: a smoker, a former smoker, a nonsmoker, or a never-smoker. We are all lung cancer patients, on

241

the same team, and we have to change our words in order to kill the stigma and save lives.

Many believe the nonsmoker angle will catch people's attention, and it does for the moment, but at what cost? Think about it. When someone is forced to heavily emphasize that they never smoked, the message being sent to the other 85 percent of lung cancer patients who are smokers or former smokers is, "You are the ones that deserve lung cancer." While I know that's certainly not the intention, focusing on stories of never-smokers who get lung cancer as a way to validate the disease isn't productive and hasn't worked in the 15 years I've been trying to change the conversation.

Anyone can get cancer, and regardless of what caused it, no one deserves to be diagnosed with or die from lung cancer! The pain from watching someone you love suffer the cruelty of lung cancer until their last breath is unbearable, so does it really matter whether or not they smoked? Does it mean that they deserved to die? Does it minimize the loss? Does it mean those left behind deserve less sympathy?

Bottom line: What matters are the faces of lung cancer; it's your mom, your dad, sister or brother, your friend or your child. It could even be you! What matters are the desperately needed research funds because advancements in treatments are helping patients live longer and better lives. Focusing on education, awareness, and support matters because lung cancer patients and their families need to believe there is hope. But, what matters the most is that the lung cancer community stands united as one team with one voice!

Let's show our faces, share our stories, and humanize the disease. Let's stop talking about smoking and start talking about lung cancer. Let's change those three words to *I am sorry* or *Can I help*. We need words that help instead of hurt.

Let's kill the stigma and save lives.

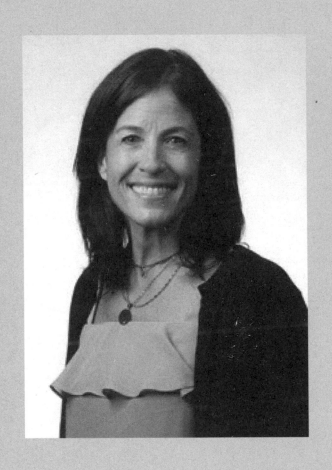

18

Jill Feldman

Jill Feldman was there at the very beginning of lung cancer advocacy, one of the original board members of the LUNGevity organization in 2001. Jill's passion sprang from the fact that both her parents, two grandparents, and an aunt had all succumbed to the disease. Among the six women and one man to establish LUNGevity, though, she was the only one *not* suffering from the disease herself.

At least not yet.

"I decided I was going to be my own advocate," she recalls. "I didn't want my four kids to ever go through what I had gone through, so I began having scans when my mom was diagnosed. All was good until 2009 when, at the age of thirty-nine, the unthinkable happened and I was diagnosed with lung cancer and became a patient myself."

As incredible as it may seem, yes, you heard that right.

"I had no control over my losses, but the attitude in how I dealt with them was my choice—I chose not to be a victim, rather a messenger. With that simple realization, I have worked hard to raise awareness

245

and money to fund lung cancer research, and doing so has also helped me make sense of all that I have been through. There have been more advancements in lung cancer research in the past seven years than in all of the previous thirty. I have options that my mom, dad, and so many others didn't, like targeted therapy and focused radiation."

Jill is speaking to me from a summer camp in Indiana, where she spent the summers of her youth. It's her respite, her escape, a place where time seems to stand still and the pace of the world can be slowed to crawl. A place where bad things and thoughts stay out, even cancer.

"My dad died May 3 in 1983. Six weeks later I was going back to camp. I didn't want to go, but my mom said, 'When you go to camp, you get away from what's going on outside camp. It's predictable. It doesn't change. Nobody has to know what you've gone through unless you want to tell them.' And she was right. I was able to escape reality, and every summer after that I've been able to escape too. When I returned as a counselor while in college, I wasn't really escaping anything at that point, but it felt comfortable. It felt like home. Brought back that sense of comfort."

Jill has remained a counselor virtually every summer since, returning as a full-fledged adult, and mother, so her three daughters could attend the camp at reduced rates. Her son never attended because it just wasn't for him, something she's fine with.

"It's like a fountain of youth where nobody and nothing changes. My doctors had a rough time when I told them I was going to camp and that all my scans and tests needed to be scheduled accordingly. Nothing was going to disrupt my summers there, and it was the best thing in the world for me."

An outlet, in other words, a place where cancer is rendered a mere part of Jill's life, if that. There's a lesson there I've learned from other lung cancer patients as well. We all need something to lose ourselves, and our cancer, in. Call it our happy place or anything you want, but it's what we see when we close our eyes during a chemotherapy treatment or a follow-up scan. Many lung cancer survivors turn to advocacy.

Others maintain strong presences on social media. Others take up a sport, or replace an athletic endeavor they're unable to do anymore with a new one. For Jill, it's summer camp. The key is to find something, anything, where you can go physically, in your mind, or both where the cancer can't follow. And that helps you in so many ways because it assures that your life is about more than just your disease, the next scan, or the next treatment. And when you look cancer in the face again, you're much better equipped to stare it down.

"I wrote this blog not long ago," Jill tells me, "about these three different patients who left little, little kids behind. It was so painful, and people are always asking why I put myself through that, through the emotional toll it takes. 'How can you become friends with someone you know you're going to lose?' they ask me. I quote them a song title from the show *Wicked*, 'Because I Knew You,' because I got to know them and it was worth it."

Jill's story is so unique, even in the lung cancer community, that it's sometimes hard to know what to say to her. There are no answers or easy explanations about how one family could be so riddled with lung cancer, or any cancer for that matter. I can't even imagine the odds of a person losing their parents, two grandparents, and a beloved aunt all to any one single disease, only to contract that very disease themselves. It's utterly unthinkable, Jill's disease having taken a different kind of toll on her four kids than the loss of both her parents to lung cancer took on her.

"Imagine, I always say, imagine what it feels like to be diagnosed with the same disease that I literally watched kill my mom and dad. My kids never got to know my parents. I was thirteen when my dad died, twenty-eight when my mom died and three months pregnant with my oldest daughter. Then all of a sudden, eleven years later, I get diagnosed. It was surreal. Okay, you think, come on; if my life were a movie, people would have walked out because it was all so unbelievable. I was president of LUNGevity at the time, and I don't remember including that in the marketing plan. This doesn't happen in real life.

And what made it even harder was that my kids associate lung cancer with death. Everybody who gets it dies, because everyone in our family who got it died. My kids were twelve, ten, eight, and six when I was diagnosed, and I thought, *Oh my gosh, I know exactly how they feel.* I remember my innocence being stolen. I remember anger, fear, thinking that my life was ruined. Why did I have to be that kid?

"So knowing what I went through, I was extra sensitive to my kids in how I gave them information. When I was diagnosed, I didn't tell them anything until there was a plan in place, and then we didn't do it in a group setting, some kind of family meeting. I told them individually. I told my son during a car ride. I told him the cancer was gone for the first time, that the surgery had gotten it all, in another car ride.

"'Is it going to come back?' he asked me."

"I said, 'Jack, are you ever going to break your leg again?'"

"'I sure hope not.'"

"'But you don't know. You can't be sure.'"

"My youngest daughter had the strangest reaction. She'd suffered through a chronic disease herself, and she didn't want to go near me for months after I told her. She wanted nothing to do with me, and she'd always been so attached to me because I'd been her caregiver when she was sick. I remember when my husband brought the kids to the hospital, she wouldn't come into my room. But I never took it personally. You can't."

Jill is highlighting another common occurrence around families that are struck by lung cancer, that being that no two reactions are necessarily alike when it comes to kids. You just don't know how children are going to respond. We've seen in these pages how often children take on the role of de facto caregivers—not because they have to so much as because they want to. But it was different for Jill because her kids had grown up with lung cancer well before she was diagnosed. They'd heard about their grandparents and their aunt. So the disease had already struck very close to home before it came knocking on the door yet again.

"You learn a lot about yourself as a patient over the years. I'm doing okay now. I started a new treatment in May after a PET scan confirmed some growth, progression, in November. I dragged my feet on it, didn't want to overreact. My thinking was maybe we had a choice with targeted radiation, that we could go after the most aggressive spots and leave the others alone for a while. I wasn't willing to give anything up and I was traveling a lot at the time, all over the country. I'm struggling with this for the first time in a long time. For all these years, this disease has beaten me down time and time again. It's emotionally exhausting, but I refuse to let lung cancer interfere with my life. And on top of everything else, I'm worried that my kids were having to go through the same thing I did when they were my age, and I hated putting them through that.

"It's taken me a really long time to process the whole thing. It's all about needing to figure out the right mindset. Physically, I have no control, but mentally I do. And having some control and not allowing the disease to beat me down mentally is why I'm always able to rally. I'm just not going to let lung cancer take anything else positive from my life and steal my joy. But I'll tell you this. For the first time since I was initially diagnosed, the one thing I wasn't overcome with this time was fear. That's how far the research has come. It's reassuring. I take this pill every night, because I'm positive for the EGFR mutation. AstraZeneca made this drug for people who suffered progression on the other ones. And the drug has proven so durable for those with progression that it was approved for first-line treatment a year ago. I think about my parents, my grandparents, and my aunt and wonder if these drugs had been available back then, at least my parents and aunt might still be alive today, just like I am after all these years."

That's a big deal for Jill, given the passion for advocacy she's maintained for over twenty years now, a stretch made even more unusual by the fact that, especially back then, just after the turn of the twentieth century, lung cancer patients weren't living long enough to become advocates. And even if they wanted to, there was no vehicle through which they could do so because the stigma associated with the disease was even more prevalent then, just as the treatment options were far fewer.

"I never actually met an original founder of LUNGevity named Gayle Levy. But I remember hearing a story about her that has stuck with me until this day. She was hospitalized, likely never to leave that room again without a ventilator tube. She couldn't speak, so she was writing in marker on this whiteboard to make her thoughts known. Gayle fought the disease until the moment she took her last breath. And now I've become the beneficiary of what I had a front-row seat watching come into existence, as a victim of the very disease I'd been advocating so fiercely for. Like I said, it was surreal, made me want to say, 'I'm sorry to interrupt this crisis, but this is an incredible moment, because I'm alive and part of the research I helped create.' We finally had momentum going in the right direction. I don't really know how to put this into the right words, but in the beginning it was all blood, sweat, and tears trying to get anyone to care or reach into their wallets to become a sponsor. Then watching the donations multiply and grow—it was amazing. And it's the reason I'm still alive. Whenever I feel defeated in my own advocacy efforts, I remind myself about Gayle Levy continuing the fight from her hospital bed.

"When I first got treated, though, there were all these researchers who had started around that same time. Most were gone within a year. They didn't choose to leave lung cancer; they left because no one was funding them. They didn't have the money. That was an aha moment for me because I knew we had to do more. Now these young, up-and-coming researchers are staying in the lung cancer community. But back then there were no walks, fundraisers, support groups, organizations, no lung cancer community. And the other reason, the biggest reason of all, was that we didn't have any advocacy because people like my mom and dad died three and six months after they were diagnosed. Even if they'd lived longer, they were too sick to have any quality of life. So much is different now, and I've been lucky enough to have had a front-row seat for the whole thing."

"It's interesting," Jill tells me over the phone from her cabin amid the pine and elm trees at that Indiana summer camp, "but at first I never used the word 'hope' in the same sentence as lung cancer because I didn't have any back when I was first diagnosed. I never did until three or four years ago when I started feeling this undeniable sense of hope permeating my life. So I got this tattoo—I'll take a picture and send it to you—that says HOPE. And it's more than just hope for finding a cure for lung cancer. It means hope for research, for the continued excitement and passion researchers have, and hope that we'll be able to raise more and more money to support their efforts."

I finally get around to asking her what she does at camp, figuring it must be arts and crafts or something like that.

"I'm the director of rifle," Jill says. "I teach kids to shoot. It's what I've always done here. I built the program from back when we had these awful, old, and poorly kept rifles. Kids would ask me how to hit the bull's-eye, and I'd tell them they needed to aim three inches higher on the target. One of the camp families heard about a child with attention deficit disorder who found herself on the range. They were so excited about what I wanted to do with the program that they donated equipment and we were able to reinstate the marksmanship qualification program that had gone away for years. And within three years, rifle became the second most popular class in camp. A couple of years ago, in one session we had seven hundred and fifty campers, and five hundred of them put rifle down as their first choice. Someone else donated more rifles and the camp received a fifteen thousand-dollar donation to expand the range so we could fit more kids. I have a camper who became a junior Olympian and these twin girls who told their parents they wanted their own rifle for their twelfth birthday. As for those who cringe when I tell them I teach rifle at camp, it's a sport and the rifle is a piece of equipment, no different from a lacrosse stick, a tennis racket, or a baseball bat."

I can't help but see her summer avocation in metaphorical terms. Teaching kids to aim for the bull's-eye at the center of the target the same way targeted therapies have kept her cancer at bay are keeping her alive. Hitting a different kind of bull's-eye. Meanwhile, Jill speaks with the same passion about teaching marksmanship at camp as she does when advocating for lung cancer. You can hear in her voice how important this place is for her. I'm reminded of a passage in a wonderful book I once read, *The Tongues of Angels* by Reynolds Price, which glorifies just that kind of experience for its hero at a North Carolina summer camp back in the 1950s.

"With open eyes I thought my way back through these weeks. And at that moment there, the weeks and their contents seemed to become what I hadn't let myself realize till now, an unspoken blessing. The one word *healing* kept coming to mind. I remember, after maybe ten minutes, saying to myself a thing that seemed directly inspired, not just a wish—*The power will follow you for long years to come*. I wasn't about to look the power straight in the eye and give it a name. But I knew I'd felt it always. And as I said, I knew then and there it wouldn't leave me. So far, I was right."

Camp is Jill's respite, her escape, the place where she goes to heal. Or keep healing. The setting insulates her from the outside world, and the outside world, to some extent anyway, includes the cancer she's been living with for ten years now. And that insulation doesn't just surround her, it encompasses the whole camp. Imagine teenagers going two, four, or six weeks without their cell phones. Jill has hers, of course, and she just received some bad news about the health of one of her friends in the lung cancer community.

"I was thinking how it's different getting news like that here instead of at home. It's just as devastating, but I'm out of context. I have a routine and responsibility here that has nothing to do with lung cancer. People know I have it, but it's not part of my identity, doesn't define who I am. At home I'm much more consumed by everything—my own feelings, social media, and up here I can't just take off and go to see my friend the way I normally could. No matter how much lung cancer consumes my life, this place remains my escape."

And this past summer (2019) Jill was awarded Staff Member of the Year. As her twenty-year-old daughter wrote in a Facebook post at the time, "Most people who know my mom know her as a lung cancer patient and advocate. But there's a whole other world where she spends two months in the summer and makes a difference. My mom was a camper at Culver, worked there in college and has been working there again for the past 8 summers. My sisters and I always say that we don't understand why the campers love her so much, but the truth is it's because she honestly loves and cares about ALL of them. Camp is her escape from lung cancer, but that doesn't stop her from making a difference in so many lives."

Unfortunately, Jill wasn't there when the announcement was made because she was on the other side of camp attending an end-of-summer celebratory dance commemorating another daughter's final year of camp, something her older daughter went on to lament in that same Facebook post.

"After a tough past six months, seeing her campers so excited would have made her so happy," she wrote. "But, it doesn't take away from the fact that both campers AND staff voted for her."

Nor does it ease the burden of the progression that has made the past six months so tough. Jill tells me that her kids took the diagnosis of her most recent recurrence especially hard.

"They were pretty upset. I dragged my feet for so long because I didn't have all the information and kept putting off telling them. I said, 'Why are you guys so upset this time? You knew this was going to happen. You knew there were these things growing in my lungs. Sure, I was pretty stable for two years, but the cancer was always still there.' The cancer wasn't going anywhere, I told them, but neither am I."

But an even darker moment followed her second surgery three years after Jill's initial diagnosis when the post-op scan showed more cancer.

"My poor family. How many times does one family have to helplessly watch lung cancer physically and emotionally destroy someone they love? I felt horrible and sad for my husband, Jason, but the worst was the fear I had for my four kids, then nine, eleven, thirteen, and fifteen. What did it mean for them, and will they face the same path I did? For a long time, I could barely look them in the eyes thinking that despite being my own advocate, my kids might very well go through what I did, losing a parent at a young age. I felt defeated and I was tired, tired of fighting lung cancer. I was in a bad place for a long time, and I couldn't figure out how to live with the fear and not allow it to consume me."

Her own advocacy efforts have helped immeasurably there, but even that comes with limitations due to the burnout she experienced from going at it 24/7.

"So I took a break. Then I realized lung cancer doesn't take breaks, so I had to get back into it right away. I tell fellow advocates, or those who are just starting down that road, to do what energizes you, not depletes you. You want to help, but what you do has to help you in a positive way too. Everybody needs an escape that has to come before the lung cancer as a priority, be more important than lung cancer. But the good thing is there are more and more advocates every day who serve this cause. Social media has been life-changing for lung cancer patients. None of us could do this alone."

Having been born into a family so struck by lung cancer, Jill struggles with whether her kids should have preventative screenings and, if so, at what age. Like so many others in the lung cancer community, she looks forward to the day when lung cancer becomes a manageable disease. She never mentions the word "cure," but she is adamant in her desire to see lung cancer get the respect, attention, and compassion other cancers receive, along with the funding it will take to continue taking leaps and bounds down the road of treatment.

"It isn't about the diagnosis but what happens afterward, how you move forward. You just cannot allow cancer to run the show. I am a realist. I'm not looking for a Hail Mary pass; I'm just looking to get the next first down."

UPDATE ON CORONAVIRUS AND LUNG CANCER

I would be remiss if I didn't cover the potentially devastating impact COVID-19 has had on all cancer patients. It's absolutely vital that cancer patients in general, and lung cancer in specific, educate themselves on how COVID potentially affects their respective treatments. Here is a primer that lays out the basics, but all cancer patients should consult their physicians and make sure the information they receive is absolutely up-to-date.

As of February of 2021, we are approaching thirty million cases of COVID-19 and over 500,000 deaths in the US alone. In this update, we want to shift our attention to another looming health care crisis resulting from the pandemic, namely a *significant decline in new cancer diagnoses*. Given the importance of maintaining appointment schedules, we will also present questions that you may want to ask your health care provider in advance of visits to the doctor. Finally, we will highlight ongoing advances in lung cancer research, because cancer doesn't stop and neither do we.

What is the impact of COVID-19 on new cancer diagnoses?

In the early days of the pandemic here in the US, many stakeholders conducted various modeling simulations to look at the short-term and long-term impacts of the pandemic, particularly related to people continuing to get their recommended cancer screenings (mammograms, colonoscopies). These studies highlighted a looming crisis, predicting a rapid decline in the number of new cancer diagnoses. Dr. Ned Sharpless, director of the National Cancer Institute, highlighted some of this data in a recent presentation at the AACR COVID-19 and Cancer Conference and in an editorial for *Science*.

A recent study showed an alarming overall drop (46 percent) in new cancer diagnoses across six different tumor types, including lung cancer, for the period from March 1 to April 18, 2020.

Additional reports from the across the country indicate an even higher drop in new cancer diagnoses. The COVID and Cancer Research Network reported a decline of 74 percent across twenty sites in the US for April 2020 compared to April 2019.

While people were encouraged to delay these essential screenings during the spring, we know that early detection of cancer is critical for achieving the best outcome and so we want to stress the importance of keeping up with your medical appointments and recommended screenings. To that end, we want to empower you with a set of questions to ask your doctor in advance of any visits so that you feel they are taking appropriate precautions to ensure your safety.

What should I ask my doctor about what they're doing to keep me safe?

It's not unusual to be concerned about the risk of exposure to coronavirus when you go to a clinic or hospital during a pandemic. A facility that is currently experiencing a large volume of COVID-19 patients, or limiting certain procedures or services, may have limitations on which patients it can accommodate. However, most facilities are ready to welcome patients.

Hospital and clinic facilities are taking extra precautions to keep their patients safe. Many facilities are posting videos and information on their websites explaining which precautions they've implemented.

If you can't find information online about the facility you want to visit, call the facility and ask about their precautions. Here are some questions you can ask your care provider or facility before an in-person appointment:

- Can the care provider conduct the visit via telemedicine? (This option requires a patient who doesn't need an in-person consultation or procedure *and* who is comfortable with and has the equipment for conducting video meetings on a computer or smartphone.)

- Can prescriptions be acquired through home delivery, mail order, or curbside pickup?
- Does the facility require everyone to wear a face covering at all times?
- Does the facility direct patients who have COVID-19 to specific entrances or areas to minimize contact with other patients?
- Does the facility screen all staff for typical COVID-19 symptoms before they start their shifts?
- Does the facility have screeners at patient entrances to ask about known COVID-19 symptoms, take each visitor's temperature, and ensure appropriate face coverings are worn (and provided, if necessary)?
- Does the facility limit nonessential companions for each patient to no more than a single individual who is free of known COVID-19 symptoms?
- Does the facility promote physical distancing through use of protective barriers, markers on the floor to indicate where to stand to stay six feet apart, and separating seats in waiting areas?
- Is each piece of equipment and appointment area cleaned between each use by a patient?
- Do enclosed treatment spaces (like MRI machines) have a waiting period between patients?
- Does the facility adhere to stringent and frequent cleaning protocols, especially in high-touch areas?
- Does the facility allow visitors in patient rooms? If so, does it require them to check in at a nursing station or other screening area before entering a patient's room?

Additional steps *you* can take to help keep yourself safe before, during, and after a visit inside a hospital or clinic include the following:

- Don a clean face covering before entering the facility, avoid touching it or your face during your time in the facility, and keep it on at all times unless a health care provider asks you to remove it.
- Wash your hands frequently. Bring hand sanitizer with you (just in case).
- Before meeting your health care provider, wash your hands or use hand sanitizer.
- When you get back to your car or your home, remove the mask carefully by touching only the ear loops. Use hand sanitizer after removing your mask.
- To be extra cautious, wash your hands and face covering and change your clothes when you get home. You might even take a shower. Wash the clothes you wore to the facility.

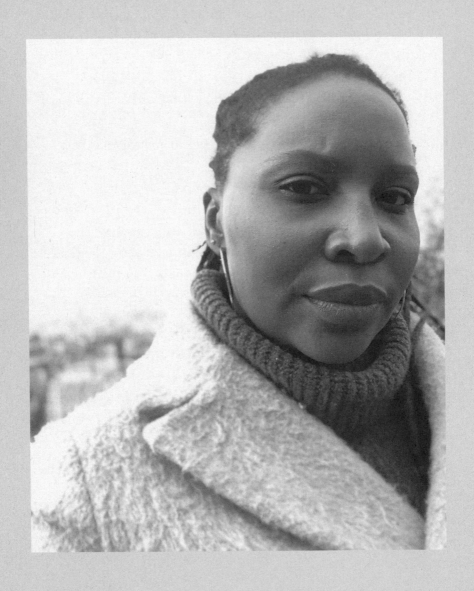

19

Brandi Bryant

On her one-year "cancer-versary," Brandi Bryant published a list on her blog, not of what she wanted to do but of what she had already done in the year since her diagnosis.

- Went on two Disney Cruises with my kids!
- Saw Beyoncé and Jay-Z in concert with awesome floor seats, thanks to my awesome soon to be brother-in-law and baby sister. Thanks, y'all!
- Went to Ft. Lauderdale/Miami and had some fun with my family.
- Saw *Hamilton* with friends and then with two of my daughters. It was SO great seeing their faces after listening to them sing the songs for months. Brought pure joy to my heart.
- Attended my grandmother's 90th birthday celebration.
- Surprised my baby sister at her Vegas bachelorette party

- Got to make birthday waffles for all of my kids and watch them reach another milestone.
- Turned 40!
- NED (No evidence of disease)

In my mind, that's a pretty busy year for anybody, much less someone suffering from stage IV lung cancer. But that's the kind of person Brandi is. In preparation for our conversation, I read all the entries from her on-and-off-again blog, and it echoes almost verbatim the explanation she gave me for cramming so much into a single year.

"You've got to live your life, seriously live your life as if tomorrow won't be coming," Brandi tells me in a phone conversation arranged by the cofounder of the GO2 Foundation, Laurie Fenton Ambrose. "Treat people as if no day is guaranteed because—you know what?—it's not. Don't be totally reckless, but be kind of reckless and a little irresponsible because that's *living*. What I mean is don't wait for tomorrow to do what you want to do. Make it happen *now!*"

Of course, by far the most important of last year's accomplishments was the final one: no evidence of disease, or NED. And that fact alone has helped Brandi embrace her new outlook on life. As she explains it, "There is some stage IV lung cancer trying to take up some space in my body, so I'm working on getting rid of that."

Spoken almost like an afterthought, because she has turned to other priorities.

"Right now, it's like everything fell out of the cupboard and now I'm trying to put it all back, but maybe not in the same place," Brandi continues from the Atlanta suburb where she lives. "I want to focus more on all these things that matter the most, more than I did before. I'm thankful for this time, this gift, and I want to make the most of it. All of these things that I put off, saying eventually we'll get around to doing them, I'm not putting off anymore. If I have to put it on a credit card and put off paying for a year, that's what I'm going to do. The great trick life plays on us is that we're always going to be here, but we're not. I'm much more in tune with that reality now. Having lung cancer has made me focus on getting things done and not delaying. Making memories. Starting life transitions, letting go of things. Focusing more on the things I like to do. I think it goes back to even before I got diagnosed. My divorce had been finalized one month earlier, and I was looking at all these changes in my life. I was ready to start fresh. Then, *boom*, lung cancer came and tried to knock me out. But it didn't. So now I'm trying to get back to that person I was looking forward to being prior to my divorce. Cancer kind of distracted me."

It's easy at times to define lung cancer patients strictly by their disease. But, like Brandi, we all had a life before we got sick, and we're going to have one afterward. And that life makes few concessions to the toils and challenges thrust upon us by being afflicted with a life-threatening disease. Imagine adding that to all the worrisome anxieties that keep you up at night and you'll have a much clearer picture of what lung cancer patients find themselves dealing with every day.

For Brandi, writing a blog became great therapy, a catharsis whereby she was able to slay her inner demons in ink rather than blood.

"I started sending my blog to my therapist, and she said, 'You should keep doing this.' After my initial diagnosis, I was searching for connections, someone who could lend meaning to this, at least make sense of what I was going through."

Her fervent quest led Brandi to the blog "Life and Breath: Outliving Lung Cancer," written by someone named Linnea, whose thoughts seemed to mirror hers at every turn.

"Last week I spent two days at pharmaceutical companies in Cambridge, MA (a mecca for pharma) describing my personal experience with cancer and clinical trials," one of Linnea's recent entries began. "As an advocate/activist for lung cancer, I continue to represent the viewpoint that those of us in clinical trials should be treated with deference and respect. That words such as 'compliant' and 'noncompliant' should just go away. That we be compensated for our time just as healthy volunteers are. Perhaps most importantly, that no one lose track of the fact that we are human beings, who are enrolling in medical research not because we want an advanced degree in community service, but rather because we are hoping that these experimental therapies will extend our lives. As people, it is our right to assume that we will not be subjected to a plethora of non-clinically indicated testing—we are more than our tissue. That we are pleased that our contribution will help others but that it is not and should not be our primary onus. We, like everyone else, wish to live. And we want to do so with dignity and respect."

Brandi had found in Linnea a kindred spirit, a kind of lung cancer doppelgänger who expressed in words much of the anxiety she was experiencing.

"She was an inspiration to me. I realized that in scouring all these blogs I was looking for anyone I could connect with. We actually met at a few conferences, and that made me want to be that person for somebody else—especially as a black woman because there was no blog for us. Because I worked on public health communications as part of my career in publication management, I kind of knew the territory. And my immediate concern was for the people who don't have the kind of access to information that I did. Statistically, I know that African-American women getting diagnosed are out there, and my concern was whether or not they knew what to ask for, like biomarker testing. I think the tendency when you get told you have lung cancer is to go into a shell because no one wants to admit they've got it. Maybe that's heightened in the African-American community because of the smoking stigma."

I remind her of the general perception that African-Americans do indeed suffer from a higher rate of smoking than whites. Statistics, though, simply don't bear that out, placing Brandi in a unique position to speak to an entire underserved population who may not know the right questions to ask or where to find the answers. But she doesn't see herself as a crusader. Not at all.

"You're diagnosed, you're in shock. You want to know what your plan is going to be. You want to just tell the doctors, 'Fix me.' Early on in my being diagnosed, after I tested positive for ALK, I was looking at receiving either targeted therapy or immunotherapy. I knew from a Facebook group I'd joined, the information contained there, that targeted therapy might not be the best option for me. And I just want people to know what I know, know more than me. I don't want people to be as shocked at every turn as I was. I want to be there for them the way organizations like yours were there for me."

I was a fifteen-year lung cancer survivor at the time of our call. As of our first phone conversation, Brandi was going on eighteen months. More than just duration, though, separates us, and the simple fact remains that while no two lung cancer patients are the same, they can all benefit from the right information and advice gleaned from the kind of experience Brandi and I now share. Her ALK-positive diagnosis made her a prime candidate for a targeted therapy that she was able to take after she progressed while being treated with chemotherapy and radiation. Hence that cancer-versary list that opened this chapter and the message contained in Brandi's words above that mirrors the message of this book: having lung cancer is not about learning how to die, it's about learning how to live.

"Living in the now," Brandi agrees over the phone, and I can picture her nodding as she says it. "But I was also amazed at how people overwhelmed me with kindness. Friends, neighbors, and people from my community were still bringing my family meals six months after I was diagnosed. They were still there, never left, and just wanted to know what I needed. 'What can we do for you?' they still ask me. That's priceless, and I think it gave me the faith I needed to keep going as much as anything else. I can't tell you how many close friends I've made because of this cancer. People I'd barely ever said hello to before who were there to help me when I needed it the most, even when I hadn't asked for any help. At work, my coworkers picked up the slack. Sure, the fact that I work from home helps tremendously, but there were days when I didn't have the strength to get up or down the stairs without assistance."

That outpouring of help energized Brandi all the more to become an activist and advocate for a community she'd never signed up to be a part of. As a mother of four—a five-year-old son, nine- and ten-year-old daughters, and now a seventeen-year-old stepdaughter she considers "still mine"—she has focused the bulk of her efforts on how best to address the demands and costs cancer extracts on a family, particularly on the children. She offers as an example a picture book that takes young children through the radiation process.

"The idea for that came from the Tree House Gang, a child and teen support group based right here in my native Atlanta. I want to take that principle even further. Explaining what the new cancer treatments look like to children, maybe a book about moms that tells how we're healthy but we're also not healthy. Women are getting diagnosed younger and younger with younger and younger children, like me. I feel sad that my youngest only knows his mommy as being sick. He knows I'm better, but then he sees me taking pills and asks, 'If you're better, why are you still taking medicine?' I tell him, 'It's because it makes mommy better.'"

Brandi speaks glowingly about Camp Kesem, a summer camp experience created exclusively for children with a parent who has cancer that was founded at Stanford University in 2000 and has since expanded to 116 chapters in forty-two states across the country. The camp's existence speaks to the ripple effect on kids when a parent has cancer.

"All of my kids wanted to go, even my oldest, the seventeen-year-old. They all benefitted from it and needed to know that there's a community out there to support them too."

But Brandi has had her share of dark moments too.

"I'm sorry that I left y'all hanging," she wrote on her blog in late July 2019, just a few weeks before our initial conversation. "The truth is that I had a major anxiety block with those results in January/February. I would've met with my doctor in a few days, but I'd learned that I could get results in my patient portal. I had never needed to depend on the portal for results because I was always getting them the same day, but this wait seemed excruciating. It was like I couldn't remember how to be patient and wait for things. Anyway, I looked in the patient portal the day after my scan and it said that the results were pending until Feb 2nd. I'm not gonna lie—I logged in every day to see if I could access them. On the morning of the 2nd, I logged in—still unavailable. At that time, I told myself to just wait until the 7th when I see Dr. Pillai. It will be fine. I didn't listen to myself because my other self told me to get those damn results. It was the middle of the night and I was alone. The anxiety was overwhelming, but I clicked it. Luckily, the results were good. That, though, didn't stop the whole experience from shaking me to my core. I was already fragile but after that I started keeping everything inside, bottled up. I just didn't feel like sharing anymore. I started writing this post in February!!! Five months ago, y'all!"

A dark point, as Brandi puts it, in the midst of what should have been a high point. In retrospect, she believes the prolonged anxiety attack was provoked by clicking on potentially life-changing information while literally alone and in the dark.

"I was thinking then that I don't have a caregiver. I always have someone with me at appointments and such, but not a single dedicated caregiver. I was thinking of seeing people alone in the waiting room or chemo room and feeling bad for them. Then I realized I was one of them, because I don't have one person who knows everything that I know. I was solo, and that became heartbreaking for me in ways I didn't expect."

That feeling has served to motivate her advocacy and activist efforts all the more, her therapy becoming not just about writing, but also doing.

"I attended my first conference because I had a friend who knew Chris Draft, who founded the Chris Draft Family Foundation along with his wife to fight disease before lung cancer took her life. It was five days after I was diagnosed, and I didn't even know my stage yet. But I was meeting people and learning about research, taking that first step toward believing this might be all right, I might just make it. We need hope to live and survive and thrive and be okay. I was so lucky to get that kind of education so early in my diagnosis. Then I emailed your foundation on the subject of second opinions. I wanted so badly to connect with people, especially other moms who were going through what I was so I could ask them how they did it. The not knowing scared me more than anything, even the treatment, and you told me, 'If there's ever anything you need, let us know.' So much had piled up on me, I can't describe how important hearing that was."

Now she wants to be the person looking to help, instead of the one in need—or maybe both. Maybe that's what continues to drive Brandi, because she can so relate to what those who reach out to her are desperately in need of.

"I tell them there's a lot of hope. If this doesn't work, there's something else. There are options. I tell them, 'I'm here for you. If there's anything I can do, I'm here for you.' I know how much that means."

Next on her list, Brandi plans to take all of her kids to Paris, expense be damned. She figures they deserve it.

"It's been so hard on them, especially coming so close to the divorce. We decided that we had to tell them, couldn't try to hide it because they needed to understand why everything, including their schedules, was going to change. I think one of the best things we did was tell them early, within a week of my diagnosis. My now ten-year-old daughter, who had a classmate who lost her mother to breast cancer, asked me, 'Are you going to die?' And the hardest thing for me was not being able to promise her that I wouldn't. We promise our kids so much, it was so hard to tell her that I just don't know. But I promised that if anything changed, I'd tell her.

"I was also planning like everything was going to be okay. I always map everything out, and cancer wasn't going to change that. My kids had always wanted a dog, and I thought this was the perfect time to finally get one. We decided to adopt a rescue dog. Then I saw a question on the application: ARE YOU SICK? I couldn't believe it. All I could do was laugh. What, because I'm sick I don't deserve a pet? So I skipped that question, and we got this great dog with matted hair who was some kind of Doodle. It worked out great. The kids love Bailey. I look at him and say, 'We're going to be around together for a long time, Bailey.'"

For Brandi, it's more of the same: make sure she does everything she's been putting off, from the dog to the trip to Paris. That's become her mantra.

"It's *The Power of Now*," she says, referencing a book by Eckhart Tolle about enlightenment. "The past is behind us and the future is nothing more than an illusion. All we have is now, and all we can do is make the best of it every single day."

My son Jared is forty-seven and works in the construction industry. The role of caregivers in a lung cancer or any cancer patient's life is so vital. I asked him too to share his experiences. I remain struck by how the positive effects of becoming a caregiver mirror those often experienced by the patients themselves.

Lung cancer has changed my life, my family's life, and my mom's life. That's not surprising; what's surprising is how that change has been for the better. When you see someone go through what my mom did, it makes you think about how many people go through life complaining about everything, every little thing. But when someone you love gets lung cancer, you let the small things go and appreciate everything more. The way you used to think about life, by comparison, feels ridiculous when patients like my mother are so positive about everything, regardless of their condition and what they're going through. They're so much stronger. You see something in them that you want to see in yourself. I realized I wanted to wake up every morning and be like that, look at things the way my mom does. Notice all the things every day that we normally walk right by. Be more connected and centered. It's sad that it took something like this to bring me to that place. As a healthy person, I'm just glad I got there without being sick. Looking back, I think I was searching for that for a long time, but I didn't realize it until I saw it.

I've spent a lot of time finding that place my mother got to and tried to get there too, and that's changed even the way I raise my own kids. I think about my mom, all the limitations she has to live with. Some people go through their whole lives without ever having to think like that. We went on a family trip to Europe recently, and my mother needs to take oxygen with her on the plane. When we landed, we asked if she wanted us to get her a wheelchair, and she flat-out refused. She'd rather walk five hundred feet on her own, even if it meant having to stop every fifty or so, instead of having somebody push her the whole five hundred. Tasks like that can be so hard for her, but she does them with a smile on her face.

I've seen the effect she has on people. It's never about her, it's always about the people around her, especially the patients who contact her for help. They're able to enjoy their time so much more than they would have if they'd never picked up that phone or sent that email reaching out to my mom. She empowers people when she talks to them because she's not sitting there talking about her ailments; she's pushing them in that metaphorical wheelchair she refused to use. That's what I want my kids to learn from her, that any moment things can change, so they need to understand what's really important. I want them to be that person themselves. Be that person when everything goes against you.

What I've learned from my mom is that no matter what happens in life or what you go through, there's always another way to go than self-pity. How you respond to something, adversity, is a choice, not a given. That's when she's at her best, and she's been that way her entire life, from the time she worked her way up from secretary to president of an oil company. The tougher the situation, the better she was at handling it. That's why, when faced with her greatest challenge of all, she really shined. She has the ability to connect with people, from senators and CEOs to the people who serve their meals. Everyone gets the same treatment from my mom. She sees the best in people and makes sure they see it in themselves.

It struck me on that family trip that she chose to spend the rest of her life helping others suffering from what she suffered from, never knowing how long she had or if she'd ever see the product of what she was doing. But I don't think it mattered because to her, even helping five or six people would have been enough, plenty. Whatever bad thoughts she may have had at one point, she knew other people were going to have the same bad thoughts, and she wanted to help them. And they're better people for knowing her.

My Story: Surgery and Aftermath

In less than three months—after all the scanning, poking, and testing—I evolved from "I can't believe this!" to "I'm going to beat this!"

I no longer worried about dying. I refused to let cancer rob me of my life.

I'm in good hands with Dr. Jablons and his amazing team, I thought. *I'll be fine!*

My surgery was scheduled, coincidentally, on St. Patrick's Day. My lucky number had always been seventeen. With a bit of Irish in my bloodline, I figured having surgery scheduled for that day was a good sign. My husband Tony's take was that it was better to operate early, knowing all the partying that typically happened on that day.

I arrived at UCSF Hospital with my entire family as dawn was breaking.

"Mrs. Addario, they're ready for you," the nurse said.

Tony kissed my hand. "You're going to be fine!" he said, staying by my side as the orderly wheeled me through the swinging double doors.

My girls tried to stay strong. I craned my neck back for one more look at them. Their wide eyes filled with unshed tears.

Tony squeezed my hand. I prayed.

One of Dr. Jablons's assistants greeted us. "Did you bring your scans?"

"No, we dropped them off at the office on Tuesday," Tony said. "A week ago."

"We don't have them," she said. "Don't worry, though. I'll call Dr. Jablons."

Tony doubled back to the assistant a short time later. "Did Dr. Jablons get the scans?"

"No."

"Well, how can he operate?"

"He has them memorized."

"Is he going to cover one eye and operate with one hand behind his back?" Tony wisecracked to me in a whisper.

I was caught off guard too, but I had to stay positive, not cynical.

That Dr. Jablons was willing to tackle my complicated surgery when no one else would was enough to make me believe he'd crossed my path for a higher purpose: to save my life. Scans or no scans, I had complete confidence in him.

"I'm going to make a fourteen-inch incision down your back to get to that upper-left lobe of your lung," he said during our pre-surgery chat. "It will be a standard left lobectomy. I'll take out the lobe. The other surgeons here are going to repair the aorta, once I peel that tumor off, and then repair the subclavian artery."

Dr. Jablons's team included a vascular and heart surgeon who also gave me their spiel before they took their place on this surgical assembly line.

The last thing I remember was hearing John Lennon's "Imagine" playing through my mind as I counted, "One… two… three…"

The plan was for each surgeon to step out and update the family once they completed their task while the next one got started.

"She's doing well."

"It's looking good."

273

"Everything's going smoothly."

Since I had responded well to the chemo, the tumor was practically dead when they removed it. Once they opened me up, I got zapped again—using radiation machines mounted on the ceiling.

Many hours from the time they wheeled me into the OR, I strained to open my eyes. Everything was blurred. I took deep breaths. Squinted and glimpsed the figure of my husband, Tony, leaning over me. His reassuring grin was among the greatest sights of my life.

I had survived!

ICU was too busy to accommodate me, so I had been wheeled downstairs to a general waiting and prep area sectioned off with curtains and a private nurse. Still disoriented from the anesthesia, I struggled to sit up. But something that felt like a garden hose protruding from my back made it difficult. And then I heard a commotion.

Still squinting, I saw what looked like the silhouettes of two guys in handcuffs and orange prison jumpsuits being escorted by police into a curtained stall across from me.

"What the heck is going on?" Tony asked the attending nurse.

"They're prisoners here for surgery."

"Prisoners?"

By then, Tony wanted me out of there as much as I wanted to leave.

"How do I skip ICU and get a regular room?" I asked.

When I didn't get a satisfactory answer, I had Tony help me out of bed. I walked around the floor dragging those tubes and devices behind me. It was horrible and painful. But I was desperate to get out of there.

They finally put me in a room but must have neglected to go through the proper channels

"Who are you and what are you doing here?" a nurse asked, spotting me inside.

"Well—"

"Who sent you?"

"Doctor—"

Before I could finish, she stomped off. I just knew I was about to be evicted. But I was in agony and exhausted after such major surgery and was prepared to be a squatter if necessary. And five days later, I was still in that room hooked up to machines with tubes. I lay in bed in excruciating pain, as if an elephant was sitting on my chest.

"Can I go home?" I pleaded.

"We can make that happen if the drains are clear," the doctor said. "But first, we have to take the lung tube out."

With that, the nurse braced her knee against my back, grabbed the tube with both hands, and yanked it out in one long motion, the last thing that needed to be done before I could go home. Tony helped to load me up in the back seat of the car. He cursed under his breath all the way home for agreeing to the early release. He had to take side streets at ten miles per hour for twenty-four miles because I couldn't handle the bumps and potholes or the stops and starts.

Once at home, the pain was too intense to move, so I didn't want to get out of bed or eat. Instead, I stayed under the sheets and kept the blinds drawn in my bedroom all day—reminiscent of my mother, who did the same thing so many times before she'd succumbed to lung cancer, which made the whole experience even worse.

"Come out, you'll feel better," I'd tell her, hoping it would help.

It never did.

"Come out, you'll feel better," Danielle and Andrea told me.

It didn't work for them either.

"You don't understand," I moaned.

I hurt. I was depressed. I'd lost my autonomy. I was mostly confined to bed, utterly dependent on other people. I continued to try to do for myself—take a shower, fold laundry—but my family was afraid I'd hurt myself.

"I'll watch Mom today," Andrea would say.

"You go take the day off," close friends would tell Tony. "Go play golf. Go to the baseball game. Do whatever you want. We'll make sure someone is here with her."

Tony felt confident enough one day to leave me alone while he went grocery shopping. When he called to check on me—no one answered. So he called Danielle at the boutique.

"Your mom's not answering. I'm on my way home right now!"

The girls jumped into Andrea's car and sped home too—seventy miles per hour in a thirty-mph zone. They got pulled over, of course.

"What in the hell are you doing?" the policeman said.

"Our mom has cancer! She's alone and not answering the phone."

"Wait. A call just came in from another officer about a man heading southbound to San Carlos with the same story."

"That's Tony, her husband!"

"Go on—get to your mom's house. But watch your speed!" he said.

They all arrived at the house at the same time and burst through the front door screaming at the top of their lungs.

"Mom!"

"Bonnie!"

"Mom!"

"What?"

"Where have you been?!"

"In the shower."

"I've been calling and calling," Tony said.

"I guess I didn't hear the phone ring."

After that, Tony didn't want to leave me alone anymore.

I couldn't be sedentary. I didn't push myself—no one would let me, anyway—but as I slowly became more active, I needed to use fentanyl patches for my pain. Fentanyl is fifty times more potent than morphine. Over time, the patches made me feel groggy and loopy, and that scared me.

"Enough!" I exclaimed on my most disoriented day and ripped off the patch.

On one of the few days Tony left me alone at home, he returned to find me doubled up in a ball on the sofa—shaking.

"What did you do?"

"Nothing…nothing…"

He called my doctor.

"What happened today?" the doctor asked. "Did she fall?"

"Did you fall?" Tony asked me in turn.

"No, nothing like that," I whimpered. "I just took off my fentanyl patch."

"You did what?!"

"Take her to emergency right now!" I heard the doctor order over the phone.

When we reached the hospital, the doctor put on a smaller-dosage patch to wean me off for good.

Just when I thought I was on my way to recovering, my hip began to hurt—right where it met my femur at the knee. The pain was so excruciating I could barely walk, barely move. I was afraid to tell anyone.

What if the cancer metastasized to the bone? I wondered.

I put off calling the doctor until I got to the point where I couldn't walk at all. He referred me to a cancer orthopedic surgeon at Stanford.

"You have necrosis of the hip and femur," that doctor said. "Your chemo and steroid therapies created a blockage in the blood supply to your bone. I might be able to regenerate the blood supply if I take a plug of bone out of your hip."

Thankfully, it was an outpatient procedure, but I didn't want to go home and rest afterward, as recommended. Tony was away, and I wanted to join my kids at our family retreat for the weekend.

"Can I please go up to Tahoe?" I begged the doctor.

"You can't put any weight on this leg," he cautioned. "It's too weak now. You have to let it heal."

"I won't walk up any stairs. I'll sleep downstairs."

"You'll be on crutches," he cautioned.

"Deal."

I asked my son, Jared, to drive me.

"Mom, are you sure this is a good idea?"

"It'll be good for me to spend time with you young people in Tahoe."

No one was thrilled with the plan, but they went along with it because we always had fun together and they knew it was pointless to argue with me.

Determined to keep my promise to the doctor, I used the downstairs powder room to get undressed to avoid using the stairs. As I struggled to put my jammies on, I inadvertently transferred my weight to my bad leg. I felt a shooting pain literally from my toes to my head and felt my leg crumple under me. I hit the floor, ending up stuck between the cabinetry and the toilet.

"Oh my God!" Danielle screamed, alerted by the sound. "I'm calling the EMTs right now!"

"Don't you dare!" I screamed. "Just give me a minute."

"Give you a minute? No, Mom, I'm calling nine-one-one."

"Danielle, help me put my pants on. I don't want anyone to see me like this!"

I cringed with pain as the kids tried to get me into my pajama bottoms.

"Your minute is up," Danielle barked. "I'm calling nine-one-one and Tony."

Tony might have been the girls' stepfather, but you wouldn't know that. They had always been close, but my cancer had drawn them even closer.

The firefighters showed up in a matter of minutes. They crowded into the small space to strategize how they were going to get me out of there.

"Ma'am, you're going to scream," one said, "but we've got to get you out of this position."

They gave me morphine right there on the spot.

It was 12:30 a.m., but Danielle called Dr. Marcus, who had become my primary physician. She knew I deferred to him for everything. He didn't just treat his patients; he managed their families as well.

"They're taking Mom to some hospital in Truckee," she said. "Is that a good hospital? Can they treat her there? Do you know anything about it?"

"It's orthopedic," he said. "They're well versed in handling a lot of broken-bone cases from skiing accidents. She's in good hands."

Tony got to Tahoe in under three hours, a drive that usually takes a minimum of four.

"There was blood in the vomit," the ER doctor told Tony and me, "and that concerns me."

He delayed surgery until he could determine why I was bleeding internally.

They snaked in a camera to view the surgery site. When my femur snapped, my hip had fragmented. Fortunately, none of the pieces nicked the femoral artery.

They couldn't operate until Monday or Tuesday, but by then, my leg had stiffened. They ended up putting a titanium bar down my femur from my hip, with two five-inch bolts at the knee and mid-femur and a big bolt in the hip. I had to stay in Tahoe at the hospital for a week.

Once back home in California, I discovered that my foot on that side had become crooked because I was convulsing during the surgery. Two months later I felt well enough to venture out to dinner with some close friends while Tony was off at a class reunion in Philadelphia. I was having a great time, until I suddenly had difficulty breathing.

"Please drive me to my house," I told my friend Dani.

When Tony got home, he found me asleep in the TV room.

"What's wrong? What are you doing down here?"

"I don't know. I had a hard time breathing at dinner."

"How long has it been going on?"

"Four or five hours."

"We're going to the ER," he announced.

"No! I'm done with hospitals and operating rooms," I said. "Let's just see where this goes."

When I couldn't get up to go to the bathroom without gasping for air, Tony said, "That's it!"

And he put me in the car.

I did not want doctors to admit me back into the hospital. I desperately wanted to go to Italy on our first family vacation in a very long time. My doctor had already green-lighted the trip. He equipped me with a small airline-approved device that scrubbed the nitrogen out of the air to keep me from having breathing problems if the plane was over-pressurized. I hated it, but I would have agreed to anything just to get away.

Those plans fell away the next morning, though, when the diagnosis came back as pulmonary embolisms—three blood clots that had dislodged and traveled into my lung and were obstructing my breathing.

"You're lucky, Mrs. Addario," the doctor said. "Most people die from these in as little as thirty-one seconds."

He put in a filter to keep any more clots from going to my heart and then put me on blood-thinning drugs to dissolve them. As the clots broke up, they went farther out into the periphery of my lung. Italy was out of the question.

"The rest of you go ahead," I told the kids. "Use the place and take some friends."

"We're not going without you," they insisted.

So no one went.

During those twelve months, I powered through every disappointment, injury, setback, surgery, and painful recovery. I'd been poked, prodded, sliced, and diced in so many places, there didn't seem to be anything left in my body for them to fix.

Even though I didn't always precisely follow directions from the doctors, I survived cancer because I never gave up. My journey brought with it a renewed appreciation for life that I wanted to share with others who'd been similarly afflicted by such a dreaded disease. If I could get better, if I could survive all I'd been through and all the setbacks, so could they. So could *anyone*.

I quickly learned that surviving cancer doesn't make the cancer disappear from your mind or your life. It just moves into a place where you can lock it away, at least for the time being. Even as I embarked on the next stage of my life to fight lung cancer in any and every way I could, it's always there, lurking in the shadows.

I do my best not to listen. There's too much else to hear, too many people to help. And that's where I turned my attention, my focus. Too much time has passed since President Nixon declared war on cancer in 1971 without the definitive results anyone had hoped for.

Now, though, the war on lung cancer has a new general and a family behind her committed to winning it.

CONCLUSION

The Big Thing

This isn't a book about lung cancer, regardless of what the subtitle says. It's a book about people with terminal diseases who find the courage to live. I'm so lucky because I survived, one of the very fortunate 17 percent or so, even more so for having the chance to get know all of the exceptional people you've just met in these pages. They make up for quite the diverse group, bonded by one characteristic.

They're all fighters, sharing the attitude I expressed to my doctors upon being first diagnosed in 2004, that being, "If I'm going to die from this disease, I don't want it to be because I did nothing." Indeed, each of them has done everything possible to give themselves a chance to live a long and happy life in which their lung cancer remains manageable at the very least. Like me, they've been honest with themselves about their prognosis and the revised shape their life took on in the months and years that followed.

I hadn't always been that honest with myself.

I spent the first thirty years of my life pretending that my mother wasn't an alcoholic. That my father wasn't a controlling man who scared me. That my husband, whom I met when I was just sixteen, loved me as much as I loved him and that the white picket fence around me was real.

I ended up divorced in my early thirties, left with virtually no money and feeling like life had taken my legs out from under me. I borrowed money for the first and last month's rent on a small home for my three kids and then started looking for a job. The best I could do was become a so-called "Kelly Girl," pretty much a glorified temp. I did that during the day and cleaned banks at night with my kids, because otherwise we wouldn't have had enough to eat. I was lucky that my brother-in-law and sister-in-law owned the cleaning business that serviced the banks.

Yet through all that I was happy. I grew so close to my children that we christened ourselves the Four Musketeers. We were a team. Sometimes we had hot dogs and beans for dinner, but some nights all we had was beans. We didn't care. We were safe, and that was enough. I never dreamed I was only just beginning to live the most amazing life anyone could wish for, defined by a freedom and empowerment like nothing I'd ever felt before.

So when I met my second husband, Tony, I was ready. We met at a computer company where I had finally landed a full-time job before moving on to work directly for the chair and president of an oil company. The new me, the person I'd become, scored promotion after promotion until, fifteen years later, I was named president of one of the largest independent, privately owned oil companies in the US, gaining an office in the same ivory tower where I'd started on the ground floor.

"You're a very lucky person, aren't you?" one of the people who worked for the company said to me one day.

"Yes," I agreed, "yes, I am."

There I was, a woman with a haunted past and no college degree running a company. But I knew that marked just the beginning, not the end. I knew there was something more and bigger in my future I was meant to do; I just didn't know what yet.

But I did know how lucky I was to find Tony. I've never met a more amazing person; sensible, loving, and someone who absolutely always tells the truth. We finally married, and the Four Musketeers grew to five. One day, he overheard me saying how lucky I was indeed to have found a man willing to marry a woman with three kids.

"I'm the lucky one," he said.

Then 2004 brought lung cancer to my life, an experience you've read all about in these pages. I was too busy fighting to stay alive to realize I was being prepared for the next stage in my life, that BIG THING I knew was out there for me.

For two years, I had educated myself about the disease that doctors said would likely kill me. I was able to step away from my other corporate responsibilities, including stepping down as an oil industry president, because I had the financial resources, a supportive family, and an incredible multidisciplinary medical team willing to think outside the box to enable me to live life to the fullest. I was one of the lucky ones who beat the odds. But I wondered, *What about the 1.4 million husbands, wives, sons, daughters, mothers, fathers, sisters, brothers, or friends who die of lung cancer globally every single year?* I was happy to help UCSF raise funds, but I wanted to have a more significant impact. I wanted to drive research and make a difference, not just be a check writer and event planner.

On March 6, 2006, I woke up in the middle of the night to a startling report on CNN: "Dana Reeve, the widow of actor Christopher Reeve—famous for his role as Superman—lost her battle with lung cancer," an anchor reported. "She has died at age forty-four."

"Unbelievable!" I said out loud, shaking my head. "Enough is enough!"

There is a 90 percent chance of survival if breast and prostate cancer are caught early, and in the 80s for colon cancer. But for lung cancer, the five-year survival rate in 2006 didn't even reach 15 percent and was considerably less than that for stage IV patients. That was utterly unacceptable to me, and I felt that the time had come to make good on the promise I'd made sitting in that chair during my chemo sessions to change the injustice in the way that lung cancer was perceived and prioritized.

I paid a visit to my lawyer's office that same day to apply for a 501(c)(3) to create the Bonnie J. Addario A Breath Away From the Cure

Foundation (ABAFTC). The foundation would have a threefold mission: to provide patient support and advocacy; to educate and dispel misconceptions about the disease; and to heighten public awareness of the relative neglect of lung cancer and raise money for research.

At age fifty-six, after surviving one of the deadliest cancers in the world, I knew it was crazy for me to begin to think about starting what would effectively be a new company, but that didn't stop me. I knew that if I ran the foundation like a business, it would be a success, and I started out by recruiting some friends and supporters, including Dr. David Jablons, Dr. Melissa Lim, Dr. Fred Marcus, and Dana Reeve's sister Dr. Deborah Morosini (who penned the preface to this book), to serve on my board.

This book represents the embodiment of these past sixteen years: the good and the bad, the happy and the sad, the battles won and lost forever, fought against an insidious enemy that gives no quarter and shows no mercy or respect but cowers in the face of the grave lot willing to confront it. I found my BIG THING in the injustice that is lung cancer, surviving the disease so I might help others follow that path. I give them my cell phone number and return their calls the same day if I'm not able to answer right away. We're fighting the same thing, you see, and I don't want them to lose and will do everything in my power to see them win.

And that, to a large degree, explains the 2019 merger of the Bonnie J. Addario Lung Cancer Foundation, which Tony, myself, and my family started in March 2006, with the Lung Cancer Alliance under the leadership of president and CEO Laurie Fenton Ambrose.

"We think this is going to rock the lung cancer community," Laurie said in a video we made together announcing the merger. "We are bringing our collective expertise, our passion and compassion, together to form GO2 Foundation for Lung Cancer, where we will be empowering everyone and ignoring no one."

Indeed, combining our assets and resources is all about achieving better outcomes for a higher percentage of patients, all aimed toward making lung cancer a manageable disease. We're losing too many wonderful people to let petty squabbles or politics interfere with doing what's right and best for the people who matter most: the patients. Our goal is to do everything in our power to make sure people like those you have met in these pages, heroes and survivors all, are around for many more years to come.

I refused to take no for an answer when I was seeking treatment for myself, and I refuse to let the others facing the same fight give in to their cancer. Lung cancer is the ultimate bully and, like any bully, cowers in the face of strength like that displayed by those you've met in these pages. My life's purpose, my BIG THING, is to spearhead the efforts to give the likes of Gina Hollenbeck, Taylor Duck, Sydney Barned, Emily Bennett Taylor, Jim Pantelas, Lisa Briggs, Evy Schiffman, Michael McCarty, Lara Blair, Hank Baskett, Juanita Segura, Lois Iannone, Diane Spry, Matt Hiznay, Jill Feldman, and Brandi Bryant more weapons to fight with so this bully might be rendered into irrelevance. You're already familiar with those names, but they bear repeating. So do the names Don Stranathan, Neil Schiffman, and Paul Kalinithi, heroes we lost too quickly but heroes all the same. And a hero like Larry Gershon, who emailed recently with an update on his treatment:

"Thank you for everything you have done for me. I know you do what you do for all of us who are living with lung cancer. But you have made my life better. You have taught me to be knowledgeable about my cancer. You have given me the living room and from there, great friends who support me. You have given me a GO$_2$ family. And you have honored me to allow me to join the BABES. All of these things add up to HOPE which is all any of us with lung cancer can wish to have. But best of all I have you as a friend. Thank you from the bottom of my heart for giving me a better life."

Nothing means more to me than notes like that, and I only wish more people would reach out to me the way Larry did so I could help them too. I might not be able to help everyone suffering from lung cancer, but my overriding goal is to come as close as I can. I'm finally doing what I was meant to do, and I'm humbled by the fortune in that, the degree of passion it's taken to become a sixteen-year survivor of lung cancer, an exclusive club destined to swell in membership—if not tomorrow, then the day after that.

Welcome to the Living Room, where people come to live, not die. People like me and all the others you've met in the pages of this book. Lucky people, each and every one, because they didn't let lung cancer beat them. Maybe it will someday, but they have already survived long enough to make a difference in the way the disease is perceived and to break down the associated stereotypes. And even those who didn't make it very long at all, like twenty-two-year-old Jill Costello, left an indelible mark on everyone she touched, an inspiration to us all, not just those stricken with lung cancer. They are an inspiring lot indeed, the depth of their courage and the strength of their attitude never ceasing to amaze me. Writing this book was a true joy because it enabled me to either meet or reacquaint myself with those who stood tall in the face of a storm that would break the best of us. And once the call or visit ends and I leave them, I always leave impressed, already looking forward to the next time we're together.

When you enter the real Living Room on the third Tuesday of every month, your feet brush against a mat that reads WELCOME as you pass through the door beneath a placard emblazoned with the word HOPE. That encapsulates the message of where these sixteen years have brought me.

That all are welcome in the Living Room, where they will find the hope they're looking for. Hope, after all, "is the thing that perches in the soul," according to Emily Dickinson.

And I hope you've enjoyed your visit and that the new friends you've met in this book will leave an indelible impression on you as they have on me. They have blazed a trail certain to grow longer as the months and years go on. And for those who find themselves on that trail, know that I will be walking by your side, hand in hand, toward a brighter future dominated by a single word:

Life.

ACKNOWLEDGMENTS

My deepest thanks to Evy Schiffman, Sheila Von Driska, Dani Gasparini, Eddi Van Auken (aka "Miss Eddi"), and my babes for their contributions to, and help with, this book. And a special thanks to every current lung cancer patient and those not yet diagnosed. We are all in it to the finish.